Autism: Our Journey

and Finding Happiness

By Mamta Mishra

Fifth Estate Publishing, Blountsville, AL 35031

Cover Designed by An Quigley

Printed on acid-free paper

Library of Congress Control No: 2015952095

ISBN: 9781936533619

fifthestatebooks.com

Fifth Estate, 2015

I dedicate this book to my husband,

my comrade, by his side I have

found strength and resilience

and to my dad for instilling the

value of hard work, honesty and the

power of prayer.

I Thank You

I want to thank everyone who has helped Parag and our family in our journey to face autism and to a friend who convinced me to share our story and helped me come out from my cocoon of hesitations and fears. I also want to thank all the teachers for taking care of our kids, molding them and giving them tools to be successful in life.

My kudos to the special education teachers for their dedication and hard work. I have one special needs son and teaching him is a herculean task. My heart goes out to these teachers who have so many students with various challenges. <u>To all the teachers I want to say "Namaste" which means "I bow to the divine in you."</u> I want to convey my gratitude to Dr. Larry Beard, professor at Jacksonville State University, Department of Special Education, who made time to edit this book and guide me through the process.

Table of Contents

Preface

There are thousands of books on Autism. Some relate the efforts of a parent dealing with and triumphing over autism. Some books advocate new methods of teaching styles that the teachers or the caregivers have come up with which are working for many children with autism. Some talk about alternative medications that have worked miracles. The market is flooded with books claiming breakthroughs in the world of Autism!

What is different about this book? This book does not make such claims. This book does not advocate that the teaching styles and methods that we have incorporated are the best. What this book conveys is that every family who has a child with autism has to figure out a coping system that works for their child with autism and for themselves. This book is our journey to face autism, a journey of ongoing progress and how we have found balance and happiness while facing autism. **I claim no unique innovative methods but I do claim assimilating the research based teaching methods and styles with a great deal of love, compassion, empathy, patience and common sense applications. The consistent and persistent efforts have paid off.**

The book is different because in teaching Parag, I have realized that there are many subtleties and extrapolations that go beyond the fundamental theories. These theories, like Classical conditioning and Operant conditioning, are fundamentals to behavior modifications but they are limited and incomplete. **There are many variables that effect real life situations.** I believe nature and nurture both have a role in shaping a person. The fact that Parag is processing the information, using cognitive and metacognitive processes in his life's situation, trying to problem solve and use schema or prior knowledge for his own benefit and survival goes beyond the scope of these fundamental theories. These theories have been essential in my understanding and modifying behaviors. While applying these theories, we analyze, synthesize and expand. I **have tried to amalgamate all these theories with a lot of common sense applications so that they work for Parag and us. One thing we do is talk to Parag and we explain why he does or does not need to do something. We know and believe that he understands.** There is one pertinent message that I want to communicate to all the parents, teachers and caregivers. **Please talk to and explain to all special needs children, including children with autism because they do understand.** The children with autism who are not verbal they still understand. Teach them beyond the command language that has become the norm for their instruction process. This is mechanical and it produces mechanical responses. I have seen through teaching Parag that by opening two way communication channels, I am able to reach out to him better. When I give reasons and explanations his compliance increases and his uncooperative behavior decreases. I believe talking to the children with autism enables us to connect with them and teach them more amicably.

This book is our way of tackling autism, so it is a one of a kind story. Every family who faces the challenge of taking care of a child with autism goes through lot of emotional trauma. **This book is not about that pain but how we have overcome that obstacle and come out stronger.** This book is different because we wanted something different for Parag. We wanted Parag to develop into a happy person, who is able to function very well in his surroundings. Parag's natural talents and skills of painting and making crafts have become his vocation! It is a very fulfilling experience for us to see Parag enjoy making his crafts and see people appreciating it too. The best compliment of my efforts with Parag was when someone asked "Are you the candle maker's mother?" This to me is Parag's real success!

Purpose of this Book

The decision to write this book has not been easy. In order to protect Parag and my family, I lead a very private life. I include people in my space whom I trust and know are accepting, even when they may not understand everything. These are people with compassionate and loving hearts. It has taken a lot of thinking and courage, till the need to share Parag's story, our story, surpassed all those fears and hesitations. I feel the need to reach out to people who are in the same boat as us and to let them know that there is hope and happiness.

Once I opened my heart to let everyone in, it was easy to start writing. This book has been a labor of love. I have shared the anecdotes and events that have happened. The first draft was like a monsoon rain. I free wrote the entire book standing by the kitchen counter. There were times when thoughts and memories came to me and I had to leave everything and jot them down, for they were fleeting like beautiful butterflies and I had to catch them before they fluttered away. The editing, fixing the grammar and punctuation has not been as spontaneous. I too, like Barnard Shaw, felt like writing all the punctuation marks on a piece of paper and asking the publisher to choose whichever ones he likes to place wherever he wants in this book!

I wanted this book to be simple and short, without technical jargon. After reading this book I want readers to ponder, analyze and synthesize the information. I hope it makes them more knowledgeable in understanding special needs individuals in general and autistic individuals in particular. While reading, I want readers to feel, relate and connect. I want everyone to know is that the first thing we had to do was accept that Parag has autism, and then create a system that works for him and our family. By doing so we are happier family; all joined together with the greatest force, love!

After reading this book I hope the students who come in contact with children with autism or any special needs students may see that **everyone is unique and capable**. Also to have respect and acceptance for the uniqueness that each of us has. Siblings should also get a better perspective as to why their brother or sister acts a particular way and how to help establish a better relationship with their special needs sibling. Understanding brings empathy and a desire to help. It leads to developing a unique bond with their special needs sibling.

I have written incidents and anecdotes that have happened in the past. Many times these incidents have led to teaching strategies or an intervention plan. It would be an effort well invested on my part, if after reading this book, parents, teachers and caregivers may be able to use some of the strategies that we have applied and make it work for them too. One has to understand that the strategies need to be fine-tuned according to an individual need. I do not want this book to be didactic, I want caregivers to read and take from our experiences anything of value and usefulness to them.

I want people to understand that children with special needs don't want to give anyone a hard time; they behave a certain way because of their sensory input and also because of our conditioning of their behaviors. Once they have coping skills, that is essential survival skills, and then these children can be trained to take control of their behaviors. Reduction and elimination of asocial behaviors make children with autism acceptable to the norm. Through Parag's story, I want to convey that children with special needs give back what they get. *If you love them they love you back and so unconditionally too.*

About this story

This story is about Parag and our journey to tackle autism. The irony is my name "Mamta" means "mother's love" in Hindi. I believe I am living up to it. One family member has to become the advocate for the child with a disability. In taking care of the child with autism generally one parent has to become more involved, creating a system that works for their family. This parent is like a "Sun", a vital source of energy for the entire family, keeping everyone emotionally strong, which is a very demanding job to do.

In my case, I am lucky that I could execute all my ideas because of my husband's emotional and financial support. Many families disintegrate when facing long term care for a special needs child. Our family by God's grace has come together. To have a man in my life who is there for me and our children, no matter what, is the biggest support. My husband and I chose our positions and have bravely stuck to them. My husband does the long term planning, securing our future and providing the financial support. I do the short term planning, how every single day can be happier and richer for all of us. My special education degree has come in handy not only in finding direction for Parag but in giving a unified purpose for the entire family. **We have been able to heal, grow and blossom together!**

Every family with an autistic child has a unique story to tell. This is our story. Our story is not about success but about progress, as it is still going on. This is a journey of courage, understanding and acceptance. It is a story where we have faltered and even fallen, but never given up. It is a story of patience and discipline. The beauty does "lie in the eye of the beholder." The most beautiful and successful thing that has happened is that Parag is happy and that makes us all so contented.

This story is not about Parag acquiring a diploma or certificate, from school but it is about him having a meaningful life. This is a story about having a life, where Parag is able to use all his skills and talents to his advantage. **How he can become "fit" so as to "survive." Darwin's theory of "survival of the fittest" is fundamental to our existence.** The homeschool is not just for Parag but is a respite for us because our involvement gives us the much needed coping skills. The school is flexible, ever changing and evolving as Parag's needs change.

I have put some relevant pictures in the book along with a link to short video clips, so the readers can put a face to the story. The video clips also give somewhat of a linear perspective of the progress made by Parag. Also at the end of this book there are heartwarming comments by the people who have supported Parag's craftsmanship. Their support and believing in Parag's abilities has helped him to continue with his experiments, making and improving his candles, soaps and organic cosmetics like hand creams, lip balms, foot balms and sugar scrubs.

Our story is the story of a team. I agree that we need a village to raise all children but more so in raising an autistic child, which means to have team of people with compassionate hearts. They have come together and believe that they can enhance Parag's quality of life. For them the biggest gratification is to see Parag grow and blossom. Parag and all of us have been lucky to find such people in our journey to fight autism.

Parag's story is following an alternative path, where children like him can find wholesome education catered to scaffolding them according to their needs. **Every kid like Parag has a talent that needs to be found and worked on.** They are capable of chipping into the workforce. Caregivers need to believe in their abilities. We have to hold their hand till they can walk and run on their own. Parag has come a long way and has a long way to go, as Robert Frost said "miles to go before I sleep, miles to go before I sleep."

Many people are in the same boat as us. Maybe this story will give them hope, vision and courage. It is our attitude to life that makes even a hard thing like dealing with autism day in and day out, not only manageable but enjoyable. Every day is a day conquered and if not then the next day will be. Until there is a cure, hope and focused hard work is the only remedy to this malady. The motto that I follow and want to share with every parent who is in the same predicament is a line from the Alfred Tennyson poem Ulysses: **"To strive, to seek, to find and not to yield."**

Autism and introduction to Parag

I am making an assumption that if you have chosen this book to read then you are familiar with the term "Autism" I will briefly go over some of the facts because I know as curious readers you will google for finer and elaborate details. Autism is a spectrum disorder that effects communications, social skills and behaviors. What causes autism? There is no one cause, so there is no one type of Autism, hence the name "Autism Spectrum Disorder." The researchers say that autism is caused by a combination of autism risk genes and environmental factors during the early phases of child development.

Some common signs that babies with autism display are impaired social interactions such as no or minimal eye contact and an obsession with certain toys and a tendency to line them up. They display selective hearing, for they have limited interest in their surroundings. They may exhibit hand flapping, rocking, toe-walking, twirling objects and may display echolalia- meaningless repetition of another person's words. They may shy away from touch, like hugs and kisses and they may not smile back.

The important thing to remember is not all these signs may be displayed. When a child is diagnosed with autism they are grouped under the umbrella term Autism Spectrum Disorder or ASD. They are all unique individuals and with behavioral intervention they are able to get rid of many asocial behaviors and develop desirable social behaviors. Medications (for specific autism related symptoms: anxiety, hyperactivity, depression etc.) do help in combination with behavioral therapy. I say this not by reading so, but with my experiences with Parag mainly, and working with other children with autism and children with behavioral problems.

I sincerely believe that every human being is more than what he is and what he has. Let me explain, you may be a lawyer, a doctor or a teacher but you as a being are more than that. Some of you may have ailments, but that does not define you as who you are. You have different dimensions to your personality. In the same way autism does not define a person, and he or she has to be understood as a multifaceted human being, not just as "autistic."

Have you seen a person who only knows how to love? I live with one, my son, Parag. He has autism and through raising and living with him, I know that he loves everyone unconditionally. What makes him so loving? Was he born that way or has his environment made him that way? This is an age old question of nature versus nurture.

I believe it is a combination of both. By nature he is like an eternal kid, a cherub, who is happy, once his three basic needs are fulfilled: food, clothing and shelter. The Nurture part of the above question is easy to answer. People who are in Parag's life, family, friends and caregivers love him and he gives back what he gets. After all, we are all products of our experiences and environment. However, as a parent and caregiver it becomes a tough job to protect him and keep him safe both physically and emotionally. He is so pure, so untarnished and so full of love for anybody, that it and everybody. This makes him immensely vulnerable. He does not expect harm from anybody.

Is he high functioning? Autism is a spectrum disorder and the word "functioning" means, the severity level. The answer is as ambivalent as the question. He is not severely affected, he is not totally independent, and he is able to take care of his wants and needs. Parag is a social butterfly and is well behaved most of the time, for he knows this means inclusion and fun. I feel he falls somewhere in the middle for I have seen people with autism who are more functional, for example, Temple Grandin. The Pediatrician and the therapist say he is high functioning.

To me, "high functioning" has a slightly different meaning than what the DSM-5 (Diagnostic and Statistical Manual) says. Parag is a high functioning human being. He is happy and loving. How often do we come across individuals who are loving souls and happy within themselves? That is a spiritual dimension which many of us aspire but it is very hard to inculcate, for it requires love and forgiveness from the bottom of the heart. Parag does not have to work at it, for he does not know how to hate!

Parag's diagnosis and my cleansing

The word that made my world go topsy-turvy was "autism"! Parag was diagnosed with autism when he was two years seven months old. Parag was neither reciprocating gestures nor was he repeating words and phrases. Unlike many autistic babies, he did not gain words and then lose them later. He was randomly repeating words and that too selectively. He was quiet and contended, so everyone thought that he was a "no maintenance" baby. Talk about no maintenance, I have realized autism is all maintenance, not just for the child with autism but for the entire family. It is a herculean challenge to strike a happy balance while keeping the positivity and enthusiasm in the environment in the face of autism, knowing autism has no cure at this time. To sail through life with acceptance and enthusiasm, when winds are against you is not only optimism but ultimate bravery.

We went through a rigorous process of Parag's evaluations. It involved Magnetic Resonance Imaging (MRI), Fragile x syndrome, Electroencephalogram(EEG) and many questionnaires. **The irony was that every test came out normal but he still had autism!** I thought if I got him evaluated somewhere else, the results may be different. However, the diagnosis and prognosis remained the same. So, I accepted that Parag has autism with a lot of apprehension. I started taking him to the rehabilitation center for occupational and speech therapy. The pediatrician and the pediatric neurologist had advised these therapies for Parag. This was emotionally and physically challenging. First of all, when the word autism hit me, I had not even heard about this disorder I started reading as much information on this topic as possible. The more I read the more depressing it got. There are books and blogs about how hard and painful it was to deal with autism. The fact that it has no cure made me so desolate.

Our family is highly educated, not to mention grandparents were already dreaming of grandsons going to ivy leagues. It was heartbreaking to see their dream for Parag dashed to the ground. My husband, a physician also metamorphosed from a happy go lucky man to a workaholic. He started worrying about securing the family and Parag financially. To provide for extraordinary financial expenses due to having a special needs child, Pranav decided to open up his own practice and later expand it in various locations around the Gadsden, Alabama catchment areas. Thus came along his brainchild "Doctor's Med Care." I understand that raising a child is a big financial responsibility but raising a special needs child is even more so. A study published in JAMA Pediatrics, 9th June 2014 stated that total life time cost of supporting an individual with ASD is $1.4 million in the United States and that if there is an intellectual disability then the cost increases up to $2.4 million. The problem parents face is the specialized schooling and services, which account for the majority of the treatment options which are not covered by insurance. Moreover, many times parents try to cut down on their work hours or one parent may totally quit working to accommodate their child's needs. In our case, I did not join the workforce and teach in a school system; instead I chose to run the home school for Parag. I wanted to keep the balance and harmony at home.

Physically it was beyond exhaustion to go for therapy sessions, come home and continue working with Parag. Basically, I was thinking that I could make Parag normal. Who said ignorance is bliss? It is a scary and most unproductive use of time. I was working with Parag as a person who was obsessed and possessed but the results were at a larger cost. I was ignoring my older son, Ankur and my husband Pranav.

Before I could help Parag and my family, I had to first rise from my own ashes, like Phoenix and discard all the negativity, anger, guilt to myself and for others. I had to evolve from the "Why me phase?" to "there must be a bigger purpose for God to give me Parag." I realized that I had to face Parag's autism no matter what. **Now the choice was mine. Was I going to sulk, cry or be brave and embrace it? Choosing to face autism head on gave me an extraordinary courage.**

The biggest challenge was to block emotional pain. It hurt badly when some of my friends invited Ankur for a birthday party but Parag was not invited. Also some comments like "only one thing a woman can do right is give birth to a normal child and you could not even do that". These are just one of many examples of what I was going through. Rejection and emotional trauma created by the actions and words of people is very tormenting. My initial reaction was anger somewhat like what Timon advises Simba in the Lion King, "When the world turns its back on you, you turn your back on the world."

I worked with Parag like a person gone crazy. All the anger, frustration and rejection made me snappy, hard headed and blind. Also my obsession to heal Parag did not let me rest. I was mentally and physically exhausted. All this negativity started manifesting itself physically; I was absent minded and zombie like. Even when I was not teaching Parag, I was still thinking and making plans for his improvements. These incidents will describe my chaotic state of mind.

One day Ankur, my older son, was late for his swim practice. I was trying to get everything together and rush out with both my sons. Ankur looked at me and said "Mom you don't have a shirt on." One time I sat in someone else's car thinking it to be mine, the seat did not feel right and that made me realize my blunder. I also remember punching a phone number in the microwave. My husband happened to see this and jokingly said "come back, our children are too young, you cannot go crazy right now". His words had some magic, I believe that made me really come back and reevaluate my life.

Now I know that anger is a false strength, understanding and compassion are the real strengths. I wanted to embrace these qualities but I found out I could not get these qualities, and I had to cultivate those in my heart. With time I learned that sometimes people say and do things because they do not understand and act out of ignorance. All I had to do was accept this fact just as I was accepting Parag's autism. **Acceptance gave me the courage to move forward.** I also understood that no one can hurt us until we give them the power to do so. My dad told me a story which helped me understand this and I want to share this wisdom. The story was that when Buddha was preaching, someone started bad mouthing him. Buddha's disciples got upset and were surprised to see that Buddha was not affected by the profanity directed towards him. They asked him that how could he be calm? Buddha replied "He is giving but I am not taking." Through this story I learned the important difference between listening and hearing. I listen, an active process to the words I value and cherish and hear, a passive process to words I forget.

Once I took away the weeds of anger and bitterness, my heart started growing with understanding love and compassion. This

16

wisdom gave me the ability to compartmentalize my life, allocate time to everyone and to myself and be happy and to see the beautiful and ignore the ugly. It was an absolute about turn for me. I decided to be in the moment physically and mentally. One of the reasons for my anxiety was that I was trying to foresee the future for Parag and us. The uncertainties were making me gloomy and unhappy. I would not impress you by saying that reading scriptures and spiritual books have bestowed upon me all these pearls of wisdom. You may find it funny that these pearls of wisdom have come to me through watching Disney movies with Parag. A very important one came from Kung Fu Panda: "yesterday is a history, tomorrow is a mystery but today is a gift." I like to focus on today and short term goals, with the belief that if today goes good then tomorrow will turn into a better day. It has taken time and meditation to imbibe this wisdom. Reinventing me is an ongoing process.

Two things that I watched on television gave me immense courage and willpower in putting a brave front against autism. I saw a man with one leg climb Mount Everest. I realized that our mind has to believe and then the body can be trained to follow the mission. The second thing that I saw on the television was that the scientists had trained a parrot to do various unbelievable tricks by making it do the same task repeatedly. For example, when asked by the scientists the parrot picked the right answers for the addition of numbers and words with its beak. I thought a parrots brain is so tiny compared to human brain, if the neural wiring in the human brain is not working properly as in autism, it can be made to work way beyond imagination by repeated training! My cleansing process lead to the healing of my emotions and spirits. These two incidents from the television inspired me to the core of my soul and made me steadfast in my mission.

Wisdom from my father also has not only helped in dealing with autism but my life itself. One day when I was very distraught after Parag's diagnosis, I asked my father for advice. He said that I should learn a life's lesson from the women who carry pitcher of water on their head. The pitcher is on their head while they all animatedly talk joke and laugh. He explained that even though these women are enjoying themselves their focus is the pitcher and that is why it does not fall. He said that Parag's autism should not stop me from enjoying my life but I should always be focused towards my goal! I am so thankful for this advice because it gave me the zeal to deal with autism with all the gusto and positive energy and to compartmentalize my life where there is space for being alive and happy!

In taking care of Parag and seeing things through his eyes, I gained the gift of enjoying the simple things in life. Big happy events are far apart but small happiness is in the day to day life, one needs to see it and grab it. Parag is happy and affectionate, this rubs off. When I take Parag to the shops and when people see him smiling they reciprocate the smile spontaneously and often say, "it is a blessing to see someone so happy". He is never short of smiles, hugs and kisses. He does not need a million dollars to make him happy but a small bag of chips does the trick. I get to witness such pure love and purity of heart every day that by sheer osmosis it is rubbing on me. I know this world and worldly desires have tarnished me but seeing Parag gives me a need to cultivate as much love and purity that my heart can muster!

One thing that has helped me in the reinventing process is gardening. When Parag got diagnosed I started digging a patch of land with wearied fervor. The physical labor seemed to soothe the mental chaos that I was facing. Once I planted vegetables, tended them and harvested them, it gave me immense pleasure. It connected me to mother Earth. The saying "You reap what you sow" made complete sense. In my mind's garden I was sowing weeds of negativity and that was what I was reaping.

Gardening not only turned me from a city girl to an avid farmer but gave me a new eye to appreciate nature and I just marvel to be a part of this immense drama. My yogic moments have come by being one with nature. It gives me the absolute peace and therefore the energy and the enthusiasm to deal not just with autism but life itself.

I promised that all the dark negative thoughts will be nailed and boxed and this Pandora's Box will never be opened and peeked into for it will bring nothing but negative energy and misery. "To err is human" and I have sometimes gone back and peeked into this box and it brought me nothing but pain. So as time has passed, I have become more determined and hopefully smarter for I don't peek anymore. I am able to warn myself.

We Know Newton's law "For every action there is an equal and opposite reaction". When I read "ten percent is action and ninety percent is reaction", it had a great impact on my thought process. It is not how we take an action but what we make of it, and that is the crux. I realized that my reaction to an event is immensely vital. It helps spread positive or negative vibes. So, I try to pause, access and process and then react. It is a conscious effort to practice this every single day. This mantra has made me more positive in dealing with awry situations and it definitely turns a bad day into a very good day.

My mental cleansing has also happened through prayers. I am spiritual and believe in the power of prayers. The beauty of praying is it can happen anytime and anywhere. As I pray more and more, my prayer has evolved too. My father, a philosopher and an avid believer in the power of prayer, had told me that praying channels our positive energy and through the power of prayer we heal, find inner peace and contentment. Initially, I asked God to do things for me or better put, fix things for me. I would also pray for others and ask Him to fix things for them as well. Then one fine day it dawned on me that God helps those who help themselves. So I started actively doing something about whatever I wanted to be different. This also made me thankful for all the blessings that God has bestowed on me. Once I was able to count my blessings, I was able to deal with things with a positive frame of mind and tremendous gusto.

"My cleansing process" is ongoing, I still falter but now I can pick myself up faster. It has enabled me to live in the present. It has also given me the ability to move on without bitterness. If someone moves on without shedding the bitterness, they can never move on in the real sense because they are carrying a lot of emotional baggage. By forgiving myself and others I got rid of the bitterness and made my mind clutter free with one thought prevailing. I had to conquer autism through Parag. It is invigorating and generates a tremendous amount of focused energy, when there is no confusion! Clarity of thought is the first step towards executing the ideas! I have found out that dealing with this mind boggling Autism spectrum disorder is easier to deal with if we can think clearly. "Knowledge is power." Before we can start on the path of gaining knowledge the cleansing process is a must. Discard negativity, let the light of positive thoughts and energy in. **This is the beginning.**

Advice from the Pediatrician

When dealing with autism it is important to get the mantra down "Bite off what you can chew." When things are not short term then mental, emotional and physical overload of any kind will lead to burnout and failure. I am glad that I found this out early on.

In the beginning, I was so obsessed and possessed in getting Parag back on track that I was delving in alternative medicine, vitamins and a gluten free diet. Also, the well-wishers would come up with great new ideas and I tried to incorporate all the advice that was given to me, which meant more work for me. I started getting cranky and short tempered. I realized that this was ruining my relationship with my husband and Ankur and I was at the brink of emotional and physical break down.

I called Parag's pediatrician and to this day I believe that God spoke to me through him. He said "Mamta, autism is not like a fever that after a while it goes away. Autism is a disorder for life, so you need to change your mindset". He said "whatever is not good for Ankur is not good for Parag. For example- too much sugar is not good for Ankur and that is true for Parag too. To deal with autism the best course is to make your household as normal as possible".

This advice changed my entire approach in dealing with autism. I realized I would have to pick and choose the ideas, treatment approaches and lifestyle that will suit my family. I realized that in dealing with autism the dissipation of mental, emotional and physical energy was detrimental for the entire family. I had to **strike a balance.** I had to take a practical survival course to face the challenge.

The first change I made was giving Parag the same meal that everyone was eating. Parag resisted eating some of the things I cooked, particularly vegetables. He preferred finger foods, french-fries, chicken nuggets, chips, cookies, candies and coke. Any junk food you can think of, he loved it. Mind you he still loves them but now he loves other foods too. I became very persistent in making him try different food. The reasons for my persistence was that I had read, some autistic people are very picky eaters and they have issues with texture of food. I was so determined because I knew a kid with autism who at that time was eating french-fries and pizza only. I promised that I would not let that happen to Parag. I would not leave Parag till he ate a few spoonfull of foods that I had cooked. He would resist by spitting or turning his face away. He said "no." He cried and many times rolled on the floor, throwing a big tantrum. All this did not deter me in my mission. I remember my husband saying that if someone saw Parag this way they would definitely think that I was being mean to him. Gradually, Parag surrendered and this was a big relief. This reduced my stress a great deal, both because now I could cook the same dinner for everyone and secondly, Parag was going to eat healthy and hearty meals. I stopped giving him all these vitamins, fish oil and Secretin hormone. He takes Risperidone, for it reduces his hyperactivity and calms him down, Melatonin and a multivitamin.

Sleeping well is very important for everyone. Some children with autism have hard time sleeping or their circadian cycle is messed up. Parag too would sleep late at night and would want to sleep in the mornings. This was not working out well for me either because I would be awake with Parag at night until he went to sleep and sometimes that would be at around three o' clock in the morning. So I would be like a zombie. Parag resisted learning in the classroom because he was sleepy. Melatonin helped, along with the fact that we made Parag play outside so that he would be tired and sleep at night. I tucked him in the bed by nine o'clock at night. This way he had to lie down on the bed till he could go to sleep. Lying down was necessary. This calmed him down and made him relax. Otherwise he would be like "Tigger" the character from the stories Winnie the Pooh. Sometimes Parag does not go to sleep until late in spite of the medicine. There are days he is hyper and has a hyperactive brain, which makes him remain awake. The next day in school is challenging because the teacher has to make sure that he stays awake during the class. She may have to change the regular routine that day and take Parag for a walk in the park or to the mall. This way we make sure that his sleep cycle gets restored. Over the years I have figured out that medications help but only when they are used with proper intervention plans. Then the results are optimal.

Thus, one piece of advice from the pediatrician made me organize my life differently around Parag and it has helped to make my home into a happy and healthy household. The goal is to **simplify**, that helps conserve energy and make things as normal as possible. I also believe God helps those who help themselves. He shows the path but to walk on it is for us to do. Once the cob webs of confusion were gone, the path did not look as daunting as before. It was challenging still but there was an element of adventure. I started with renewed energy, zeal and enthusiasm.

How Home school came along

Parag started going to a day care center at the age of three. He was accompanied by an aide. Ankur was going there too. The job of the aide was to help Parag interact with children and help him participate in activities. Otherwise, he sat in the corner and was in his own world. We were very satisfied with the teacher student interaction there. In the year 2000, Parag had to make the transition into the regular school system. His resource room had twelve children with different disorders and disabilities. We were apprehensive and were doubtful as how much one on one instruction he would get. I knew Parag would not mind being left alone but then to get him back to follow instructions would be harder and not without initial resistance. We were ready to provide a "shadow" for Parag, thinking that she would be able to direct Parag into activities and the teacher would have an aide in the class. However, the school system rejected the idea. The reason given was that school system has to be fair to all children and allowing an aide for Parag was violation of that concept. The school decided to have an aide in the classroom to help all the students. We thought this was fair for all students, we sent Parag to the school, hoping for the best.

After attending few days of school, Parag started banging his head on the floor, whenever he got upset. I found out there was a kid in the class who was doing this. I was surprised that Parag had picked up a behavior so fast, for I had read that autistic children did not imitate gestures till taught. Well this one did not need teaching!

I was also overwhelmed with the paper work. The school also got a behavioral consultant to evaluate Parag. After this his IEP:

(Individualized Education Program) was set. I definitely wanted Parag to learn at a faster pace than what was on IEP. The behavioral consultant that the school had hired also gave the same recommendations, that Parag needed more one on one instructions and applied behavioral analysis would be most beneficial to him. **The recommendation stated "learning in a school setting will be harder for Parag than learning in a one to one setting with an adult only, but the school setting provides a rich and real environment for him to learn important social and communication skills...Parag requires year-round intervention. An extended school year should be considered by his IEP team".** I understand that it is hard for a school to provide one on one interaction the entire day. Moreover the school system here did not have the extended school year plan. I realized that persuading the school system and asking to accommodate Parag's needs would take lot of energy.

It was becoming obvious that Parag would not be able to be in the mainstream school system in spite of the academic accommodations. At that time he had a short attention span, mumbled randomly and he threw tantrums when directed to a task. He would bite his wrist and sometimes pinch the person who was addressing his behaviors and Parag was lacking in language.

I realized in spite of the school systems motto "no child left behind," Parag was already far behind, for he did not fit in the system that is so skewed towards test taking and memorization. Our school system is better geared towards handling students with physical handicaps than mental disabilities or disorders. **America emphasizes individuality and uniqueness in everyone. It is ironic that the American school system advocates one fit for all, main streaming and teaching Common Core Curriculum to all students.**

Is this realistic? Is this beneficial to all the students with special needs? Once these students have acquired their diploma or certificate, how many are able to find a sustainable, fulfilling job? Are there enough opportunities for them according to their skill level? The data on this, particularly for individuals with mental handicaps and autism is very allusive and equivocal. Kids with autism need training in daily living skills, life skills, and behavior management, along with emphasis in their deficit areas of social skills and communications. In general, school is not geared to teach these concepts. The school system is based on academic success which is discernable through good grades. **The pace of teaching is too fast and too vast for kids with autism.** There are many gaps that need to be filled before they can perform well. The teachers have a time crunch to finish the curriculum, so that students can perform well in class tests as well as in the standardized tests.

The problem is that in general, the kids with autism are not good at test taking. That does not mean that they do not know the material. They need lots of adaptations and modifications to be successful. The school system is not able to provide a **holistic approach** to teaching kids with autism which is essential for their all-round development and success.

I did not want to coerce the school system for Parag's needs and issues. I felt this would dissipate my energy. When you browse through the internet, you will have a long list of the rights for the parents of children with special needs . These rights allow the parents to be aware and keep the dialog open with the school system. I felt that every time I would go to the school, it would be with some concerns regarding Parag and then the school will evaluate, take their time and then decide whether these concerns were valid or not. **I knew that time was the essence for early**

intervention; I could not lose that in the quagmire of red-tape. **I did not want to pick battles when I had to win the war.**

In many states in United States of America, there are Charter or Magnet schools that are publically funded. These schools specialize in catering to the needs of children various developmental disabilities. Some of the charter schools specialize just in Autism and cater to their needs. In some states when parents are not happy with the quality of education provided by the public school system they can choose to send their child with developmental disorders or disabilities, in a private school. These private schools are equipped to provide "equitable services," or comparable services that are provided in the public school system. A "services plan" is created for the special needs student, this is similar to the IEP (Individualized Education Plan). I was not able to find these services where I live. After all this research the answer was creating a system that works for Parag and our family. Again a very brave idea but it was a precarious path, for I had to create and pave an alternative new path. It is hard and constant work, both mental and physical. I have to go on changing, modifying and building connections with people who have knowledge and experience. The biggest thing is applying the ideas and **giving them time** to come to fruition.

All these questions, thought processes and Parag's pace of learning made me decide to home school him. Before I started the homeschool, I had to be clear: what was the purpose of the home school? For us the purpose was to make Parag as functional as possible and that he should be happy. A private school gave Parag a chance to come in the class with a shadow/assistant as a kindergarten student. **An applied behavioral analyst made a by-law, this gave and allowed other students the same opportunity as**

Parag. He went to the school for half a day mainly to socialize and do his work in the classroom surrounded with other students. Parag worked at home from 8:00 to 10:00 am at home and from 10:30 to 3:00 he was at the private school. This gave him an opportunity to learn music and art, have lunch with school children, learn how to be in the queue when coming out from the class and be in the line with other children. He was accompanied by a shadow, who would sit in the classroom and make sure that class went smoothly for Parag and the other students. Parag could be removed from the classroom, if he mumbled or pitched a tantrum to resist working. The task that he performed at the school was something he was familiar with and knew what was expected of him. So the chances of his reacting loudly were rare. The new stuff and challenging skills were taught at home along with daily living skills, life skills and behavior management.

The curriculum was prepared by a behavioral analyst, who came once every month to guide us and fine tune the program. This way we were able to meet all the recommendations made for Parag in his Individualized Education Plan. Going to a private school also gave him the opportunity for social interactions in a real life setting. Parag became happier and more receptive because the curriculum was totally geared towards his needs both developmental and emotional.

For his all-round development, the private school and we his parents were working hand in hand. I am a special education teacher and a parent of a kid with autism. I see both sides of the coin. **I believe if parents and school systems can work together then kids with autism will be successful.** This will be a path of fine balance and taking responsibilities for the overall benefit of the kid with autism.

Decision to speak in English around Parag

Before we could start the home school we had to make a decision what language would be using with Parag. Our family is trilingual and we very easily switch from one language to the another. We made a decision to stick to one language for consistency, while talking with Parag. The language we chose was English because this is the language spoken in America, where he lives. Also English is a universal language. This widens his scope of communicating with people. Also, we chose that he should be immersed in one language so as to minimize confusion. In spite of our sincere efforts Parag has picked up words and phrases from other languages spoken around him and he uses them in appropriate context!

A lot of times, funny situations arises due to his bilingual vocabulary. One day, the teacher came to me and said sadly that Parag does not love her. I asked why she felt that and she said that when she went to wake up Parag, he said "shoot". To her dismay, I started laughing , I held myself and told her that she should never doubt that Parag loves her, he does not know otherwise. I told her, he was saying "shuut", which means sleep in Bihari dialect. Basically he was saying I want to sleep more. He has picked up this word from his grandma. The teacher was relieved to know this and started smiling too.

There are times when a teacher is teaching something that Parag finds hard so he says "baap re baap" pronounced (baap ray baap and literal translation is "father o father"). The intrinsic and colloquial meaning to this phrase is "oh my God". I say that when I am doing something and am flustered or rushed. It is funny that he has picked it and uses it appropriately too. I know what he is saying and it brings a smile on to my face but the teacher used to think that he was mumbling. I had to explain and now they smile too when he says this. When he says this phrase the teacher tells him "say oh my God." Thus he knows how to express the same feelings in English as well.

Another funny incident happened one day when the teacher said that Parag does not understand drinking. I asked her how she figured that out and she said, Parag says "juice pee, water pee, anything associated with drinking he is saying pee". I had to hide my smile and tell her in Hindi, we say "pi" to drinking. He is saying correctly but in a different language. Also I told her we will make sure that we emphasize the word drinking, so that he will start saying that instead. Now he says drinking instead but that does not mean he has forgotten the Hindi word. He uses it when he thinks he needs to express in Hindi. For example, around his grandma he uses more Hindi words because that is what he has heard from her. She can speak in English but he observes her talking in Hindi all the time in the house and with all of us so Parag tries to communicate with her in both English and Hindi. He has limited Hindi vocabulary but uses those in appropriate context. There are words like "de" (pronounced day, means give), "le" (pronounced lay means take) "chor" (pronounced phonetically the same way as written, means leave me), he uses them rarely because he is used to communicating in English now. Over time it has become his primary language for communication.

I remember going to a friend's house for a quick errand. I stepped out of the car. My friend came to say Hi to Parag, for he was in the car. Parag saw her and said "baaith" (which means sit-down). Parag was telling her he wants to sit-down in her house, he was inviting himself and letting her know. My friend and I laughed because we knew what he was asking. When I say children with autism are very intelligent, I witness this daily in Parag. The very fact he used the Hindi word "baaith" around this friend is because she is an Indian. He has figured out that Indian folks use these words. I don't remember exactly when he started using only English around Americans. I think this must have happened when he used Hindi words around Americans and did not get the response that he was seeking but got it from Indians, so he realized that it is a waste to use these words around American folks.

It is really surprising that he is able to comprehend all these languages, for when you ask a question, he replies appropriately in English. For example, if I ask "kha jaa rhe ho" (Where are you going), He says "potty". So what amazes me is the degree of receptive understanding. We have not taught him Hindi actively, this he has picked it up from us talking around him. It is very rare that I will ask him something in Hindi but when by default it happens, he replies back in English. He is used to responding to me in English. Parag also sings some bits of Hindi songs that he has heard.

I don't know to what depth he understands these languages. The reason I say this is because he loves flipping through National Geographic. Sometimes he will flip back a page as if he is rechecking something he missed. All I can tell is that he is able to communicate his needs in both Hindi and English. The fact that we speak English with him means he is able to communicate better and more elaborately in English than Hindi. In Hindi he is limited to words and phrases, which he has imbibed from the environment without active teaching. The amazing thing is that he is able to learn and use words to communicate appropriately in both languages. After deciding English was the primary language spoken around Parag, we had to make other decisions, like how are we going to educate Parag.

Definitions for the Upcoming Discussion

Applied behavior analysis (ABA): an intervention plan that takes into account how a person absorbs information, processes it and retains it.

Discrete trial training (DTT): stimulus, response and reinforcer. Stimulus is the instruction and the student needs to respond. Once the teacher gets the desired response she rewards the student. This is the reinforcer because it makes that behavior strong.

Incidental teaching: objects of highest interest for the students are kept out of their reach, so that they will initiate communication through pointing to the object or through a word or two. The teacher then encourages the child to expand communication.

Teachable moment: It is unplanned teaching. Learning happens organically. An example is the interaction where a mother responds to her child's curious question in the moment.

Contextual teaching: teaching done in a real life setting, therefore the term "contextual." When we take the kids to the zoo, show them animals, and talk about them, it is more meaningful because it is hands on. Contextual teaching is a combination of hands on teaching and real life experience.

Methods of teaching

I had to decide what "manner" or what methods of delivery would be employed. I decided to use Applied Behavioral Analysis as a method to teach Parag. Why did I make this decision? The simple reason is that research based data shows remarkable improvements in kids with autism through this method of delivery. "Applied Behavior Analysis has been demonstrated to be the treatment of choice for students with autism based on over 40 years of supportive evidence in improving social behavior and communication and reducing levels of problem behavior (Lovaas, 1987)."Parag's school uses **Applied Behavioral Analysis and incorporates various teaching styles: Discreet trial training, Incidental Teaching, Teachable moments and Contextual Teaching.** This took time to get streamlined but the decision to use applied behavioral analysis and gradual incorporation of various teaching styles brought structure to the school routine.

During this time (year 2000), I was also taking Parag to Walden Program at Emory University in Atlanta, Georgia every Wednesday. This is a family program that helps educate parents to increase communication in children with autism through **Incidental Teaching.** In this method of teaching the environment is arranged in such a way that things and toys of high interest for the children are put out of reach of the children, so they will initiate communication by pointing obtain that object. For example, the toys are put up on an armoire or locked away. When the kid points at the toy, the teacher may expand the pointing along with a word "give." After several trials she may add "me." This method was familiar to me for we were doing similar teaching in Discreet Trial Training. This is called forward chaining of words. We did trials where he had to just touch the objects, when we mentioned their name. This way we knew that receptively, he knew them. Then we would show the object and tell him what it was and ask him to "give me." So the major difference was that Incidental teaching required Parag's **initiation,** by pointing or through words to start the teaching process.

It was two and a half hour of drive to the Walden School. Parag was tired and irritable after a long drive, so he would not perform well there. When I told the therapist that he could do those things, like following the command "give me" and then handing the object to me, she did not look convinced. To her I must have looked like an overzealous mother who had a hard time accepting that Parag could not perform the tasks. This made me decide to videotape Parag when he was performing commands and listening to the instructions and executing them too. I made those videos over the week and showed her. This changed her attitude and she got more involved in teaching Parag. She knew he was doing a lot more than she was able to see. From this incident onwards, I sincerely believe that a picture is worth thousand words. This initiated the process of taping Parag's progress. We still collect the videos of his performance on an i-Pad. This way, when the behavioral analyst came to see Parag's progress we were able to show her his progress visually. Now, when a consultant and a veteran special education teacher come to guide us, we are able to show his progress. Observing these videos gives everyone a pretty good idea of his skill level. Based on the videos and his performance these objective observers are able to give more accurate recommendations.

I felt the need to gain knowledge and experience to help Parag. I wanted to be taken more seriously than an over enthusiastic mother. I knew that a degree in the field of Special Education would make me an educated voice and advocate for Parag. By this time I also knew that to run the home school for a long term, I needed the skills and the knowhow. I decided to go to Jacksonville State University and pursue a Masters in Special Education. This was also possible because the University is at about forty minutes of drive from the place where I live. The close proximity gave me the opportunity to run my household and take the classes as well.

Studying Special Education enabled me to see the bigger picture. It gave me a perspective and an understanding of how to tackle the behavioral challenges and teach the special needs students in general and how to approach the specific needs of Parag and his autism in particular. The education helped me to break down the skills, scaffold and create measurable successful steps and fill the gaps and reach the goals set for Parag. Taking Parag to Walden School at Emory University and gaining knowledge about Incidental Teaching also helped. I had read in an article that Incidental Teaching is not accidental. This means that the environment around the child with autism is organized in such a way that it encourages them to initiate communication.

I figured out that Incidental Teaching was a version of teachable moments. In Incidental Teaching, the environment of the student has planned opportunities to increase initiation in communication. **Teachable moments** are unplanned, the way the mother interacts spontaneously with the child. When the child suddenly asks a question due to curiosity, the mother delivers the answer and the teaching is done. This moment could become long if the interest of the child is sustained.

Both Incidental Teaching and Teachable Moments require interest from the students. Children with autism have very limited interest, particularly during the early stages of intervention. Parag too had very limited interests such as, favorite foods and toys with which he could sit in the corner and play by himself. I wanted the classroom to be more structured, so that he would also develop an ability to sit down and do a task. This is an essential ability to be able to function in the classroom and also in many public places, like sitting down at a restaurant, movie theatre or for a program. This made me incorporate **Discreet Trial Training** which is also a branch of Applied Behavioral Analysis. This method helps in creating structure for imparting drills and practice. It is based on the concept: **stimulus, response and reinforcer.** Stimulus is the instruction that a teacher gives to the student. Once the student starts responding correctly, the teacher withdraws the prompts and cues. Lastly the reinforcer is the motivator for this teaching to happen amicably.

I also felt that **Contextual Teaching** made better sense than sitting in the classroom and teaching a concept. For example, we wanted Parag to learn get his groceries. So I had set up a station with various things (plastic bananas, apples, cookies, empty milk and juice cartons etc.) with their prices. He had to make the grocery list and go to the station to get those, check the price add them on a calculator and then hand the money to the teacher. Of course the teacher was prompting and leading him in his efforts. After a while, I found it artificial and boring. I have found out that if any teaching is boring to the teacher, it is extremely boring to the students because it does not have the vitality of enthusiasm. I started taking him to the grocery store and teach him to buy groceries there. This made perfect sense because it is hands on in a real world setting. Grocery shopping had to make sense to Parag as to why he needed to buy these things. Adjoining his classroom is a room for crafts and it has a refrigerator, a microwave, a table and chair where he can eat. He makes the list of things he needs for his breakfast and lunch. On school days he has his breakfast and lunch in the classroom. He buys his sandwich stuff, which he makes during lunch or he may just warm up his ready to go meals. Parag knows that the fruit, water and cereals he is buying, are for him. Parag loves going to the grocery store on Wednesday (his day out in the community) with his teacher now he is able to use a debit card and sign his name on the receipt as well.

I decided not to use Picture Exchange Communication System (PECS) with Parag. Through this method children with autism are taught to communicate with pictures. They also transition from pictures to voice output system. I tried it for about three months and found that Parag was losing words that he already knew or he was choosing not to use those words. I felt that Picture Exchange Communication System was making him stop trying to speak. I was concerned that by incorporating the Picture Exchange Communication System Parag will eventually choose not to communicate verbally at all. Parag is able to communicate verbally and that is important to us. I realized that Applied Behavioral Analysis intrinsically incorporates modes of aural, visual and kinesthetic learning. Immersing Parag in all these methods makes him learn better because he learns through a combination of these methods and styles of teaching.

Over time all these methods of teaching are blended with the daily curriculum. It was confusing in the beginning. Gradually, all of these common sense applications came together to form the best environment for Parag's learning.

Tracking progress by a report card, maintaining a portfolio, following schedules as well as maintaining time cards, for teachers to clock in and out has all evolved over time. **All these methods of teaching have one commonality; they all require powerful reinforcers for the teaching to progress amicably.**

Materials for Teaching

Once the manner or methods of teaching were clear, then another important question arose. What matter for teaching- that is all the teaching materials, resources and tools. It is equally confusing like choosing styles or methods of teaching. There is a vast supply of teaching materials, websites and advertisements of the teaching materials eulogizing their products and claiming to have the best. The question that I faced was which of these teaching materials were really helpful for my child's needs.

I realized that spending money to buy specialized equipment to teach was not always an effective approach. I spent $3000 to buy a computer like device which was supposed to be very interactive and helpful in increasing communication skills. The device was cumbersome to operate and the voice that pronounced the words was very mechanical and not clear. This experience made me decide to make Parag use a regular computer because it is available everywhere and people will know how to guide him on that.

After buying some online teaching materials and finding them of no or very limited use to Parag, I invested in software only after getting trial sessions, demos and checking if Parag was ready for learning that skill. We use an i-Pad and a Kindle. They have proven to be very effective teaching tools and entertainment. We make sure that he has different tablets for learning and entertainment. Parag enjoys listening to his music, browsing through YouTube for his shows and watching his favorite movies on his i-Pad. The are many teaching materials saved on the Kindle and the computer. We do not want him to access it without the supervision of a teacher. It is almost like an archive after so many years of teaching. I felt that letting him use the same tablet for both entertainment and teaching would confuse him in understanding the boundaries. It is important for Parag to learn that there are certain things he should not touch or if he really wants to have them then he needs to have permission.

I also started collecting teaching material from local shops, like Wal-Mart, Office Max, local book stores and the libraries. This way if something did not work I could return them easily. Free teaching websites and work sheets are handy too. Investing in a good photocopy machine and printer has been a very good decision. We have to make several copies of the worksheets for practice. The printer helps us to printing out various worksheets available on the websites. The printer also helps us to document his performance. For example Parag has a reading program that shows the printed report of his progress for his portfolio.

The same concept is taught in variety of ways, for example-books, flashcards, three dimensional objects, computer, kindle, TV, movies, puzzles, games and music. I have seen that Parag learns better, if the teaching method is backed up with the visual and concrete hands on examples. He learns better when things make sense to him and are realistic. For example, the picture flashcards that are photographs of objects and people makes him more receptive to learning, because they are close to actual representations.

I know that technology helps us facilitate the teaching process, particularly in delivering drills and practices. **I believe that technology should not take over human interactions.** All children need to interact with people. The need for children with autism to do so is greater because through human interactions, students with autism are able to learn social skills and cues in areas they all need help with. The variety of teaching materials and worksheets to enhance a concept helps to hold the interest level. Once matter and manner of teaching was nailed down, Parag's school gained momentum.

Finding teachers and their training

Homeschool for Parag began in summer of 2000. It was very confusing in the beginning. I knew I needed a team to run Parag's school. The occupational therapist and the aide from the school system agreed to help with Parag's home school during the summer vacation. The behavioral consultant who helped make IEP for Parag also agreed to come once a month to get us started and then overview the teaching process. I also found a high school student who would play with Parag and do some skills maintenance, like going through the vocabulary flash cards, numbers, colors etc. I saw with the team in place Parag started improving at a faster rate. Once the summer vacation ended the occupational therapist and the aide returned to their jobs. I was the only one left to teach.

Hiring the right people to teach Parag proved to be more challenging than I expected. I found them through word of mouth, which was not an effective way of finding people to run a homeschool. It was disappointing to see that even when I found someone and trained them, they would leave after few months or sometimes few days. I had to figure out a better system of hiring people and also find incentive for them to stay. While studying at the University, I saw that a lot of students were constantly looking for jobs. This gave me an idea. I put flyers with the job description and a pay rate that was above the minimum wage. I distributed the flyers in the Gadsden Community College and the Jacksonville State University. This solved the problem of finding people. However, they did not stay very long.

I was looking for a teacher who could share the load of this daily teaching and impart those drills and practices. This would release me partially from Parag's school to do other things that needed attention as well. I meditated over the reason why staff left

41

even when I trained them so well. My self-analysis gave me an answer. I was at fault. I was not giving the teachers their space and authority. I would let them observe me while I taught Parag and did the behavioral interventions if a situation arose. I was always there to help even before they asked for it. The teachers were leaving in spite of the training because I was making them dependent on me! The whole approach of this training process was wrong. I had to figure out a way to relinquish my authority so the teacher could not only teach but be confident enough to handle his behaviors and tantrums as well.

So the new approach was **hands on** from the first day. I would teach a skill/task and let them do the same. I would talk about behavioral intervention strategies and what to do when needed. This training lasted two weeks and the second week was **immersing** them in the teaching and I was not in the room, I could still observe them from the camera that was set up in the classroom. I would not intervene until the teacher asked for help through the intercom system.

Research shows that teachers have a high burn out rate and this is even more so in teaching special needs students. I knew that Parag's early intervention program was very intense and I needed teachers not to burn out. I decided to train two people at a time who were going to work on alternating days. That way, if one left Parag would still have one teacher and of course me. This created a great backup system, if one teacher could not come, then with proper notice the other one could be available. This system of two teachers working with Parag on alternate days went on for five years. In 2005, we were successful with only one teacher. The intensity of behavioral interventions had diminished to the point that two teachers were not necessary.

The next thing was to make the teachers motivated. Money is a motivator but more importantly is that a teacher have ownership in the student's wellbeing. They needed to know why teaching Parag was meaningful and how they were making a positive change in his life. I made sure to make them feel a part of Parag's success and tell them how an intervention plan was working outside the classroom. This makes them see the bigger picture and how an intervention plan is working in a real life situation. For example, recently we took Parag to a restaurant and he did not blow out the candle that was set on our table. I asked Ankur to send the picture of Parag to his teacher. Parag was sitting quietly and happy. She was delighted to see that Parag was not blowing out the candle because that is one of the target behaviors we are trying to eliminate. I have mentioned the intervention plan for this in the chapter: Some behaviors we are still working on. After working for a while the teachers see the bigger picture. It becomes clear to them that they are increasing Parag's quality of life by making him more functional through their teaching and in return they get love from Parag that is so pure and unconditional.

I have found out that an education degree is an asset in teaching special needs students but this is not the biggest asset. A teacher with a lot of patience, compassion, sincerity and a big heart is! My education has helped me to chart the short and long term goals for Parag in the form of a report card and bring structure to the home school. This is important because we need to track where we want to reach by the end of the year. If I was not educated in this field, I could still get help from a professional and customize a program for Parag. The challenging part is execution of those goals through consistent and persistent drill and practice. **The special needs students benefit from repetition and Parag does too**.

The extended family of the teacher who works with Parag, has accepted Parag as a family member. They make sure that the help for Parag and our family continues. I am so thankful for their support and love. She had to leave for personal reasons so she made sure that her niece (the present teacher) was here to run the program. The high school students who are Parag's play buddies make sure that when they are not able to work for a while, like football season, they train their friend to take their place while they are gone. So the system of finding teacher has become stream lined. The people who are working with Parag are so attached to him that they make sure that his school goes on when they can't be there and they are the ones who find teachers for the school, if the need arises. They are very particular about who comes in the house. They get people whom they trust and believe that they are going to take care of Parag as they themselves have been doing.

Finding people through word of mouth was not working in the beginning but now it works. Over the years Parag's school has got the reputation of being genuine to the cause of meeting Parag's needs. They see we love Parag and very naturally they do the same. Teachers not only feel safe working here but they feel appreciated, cherished and are part of this family. Many college students who have worked with Parag are teachers now in various school systems. We enjoy being connected to them through social media and they visit Parag whenever they can. They keep in touch with his progress. So Parag's teachers may or may not have a degree in teaching but they are motivated educators.

Now, I am more of a substitute teacher. On Fridays I teach Parag, the things I teach are mainly the areas I want to focus on. . Communication is one of the target areas, so I focus on spelling, vocabulary retention, reading, maintenance of skills and anything else the teacher has asked me to help her with. If we come to a road block, then the teacher and I brainstorm to overcome it or circumvent it. Sometimes she could be having difficulty in teaching a concept. Then I try to figure out how to teach that and then the teacher and I can be on the same page with the strategies, matter and manner of teaching. Sometimes it could be that I am stuck but Parag is performing the same skill for the teacher. Then it is my turn to sit and observe the teacher because there is a subtlety in imparting of the skill that I am missing. I have emphasized before this school works because of an efficient team, all of us are team members learning from each other so that we can help Parag. It is the reason for this school's existence.

I believe when the teacher has common sense then it is an icing on the cake. This gives the teacher the ability to solve problems when they are stuck while teaching. These are ideas from our day to day lives and experiences. To teach a special needs student requires a lot of patience and people who want instant gratification and returns from their efforts while teaching special needs students will be miserable. Degree in teaching and in special education in particular is meaningless without a big loving heart!

A service industry like this requires Mother Teresa's heart in every teacher.

Early intervention: Teaching life skills, daily living skills and getting rid of some symptomatic behaviors

Some common signs that kids with autism display are impaired social interactions. For example no or minimal eye contact and an obsession with certain toys and a tendency to line them up. Also they display selective hearing because they have limited interest in the surroundings. They may also exhibit hand flapping, rocking, toe-walking, twirling objects and some may display echolalia-meaningless repetitions of person's spoken words. They may shy away from touch, like hugs and kisses and they may not smile back. Parag showed all the signs and seldom repeated words!

I left for India with Ankur and Parag. My parents and siblings lived there at that time. I needed an emotional and physical respite. I was totally exhausted and at the verge of breakdown. This turned out to be a good decision because everyone started helping with Parag's therapy. My brother took the challenge of making Parag listen to the instructions and perform tasks. Parag preferred to be left alone and oftentimes he twirled objects. My brother did not give in to Parag's tantrums; his logic was that Parag's hearing was alright. If he is choosing to react to something he wants like sound of the coke can being opened, then he is selectively choosing to listen. My brother would place an object on a chair and ask Parag to go and get it. Parag resisted it in the beginning but he realized that he was fighting against a team, and no one was giving up till he did what was asked of him. Parag surrendered and started following simple commands like "give me", "show me," "touch", "go and get".

To make Parag leave his world of lining up or twirling toys, for him to start complying and following commands was the toughest phase. It was almost like breaking a wild horse. This is the phase where tantrums were frequent and of long duration. The next phase was drilling skills to enhance his interaction with people and his surroundings. As I have mentioned earlier, Parag was randomly and rarely repeating words at this point. However, one fine day, he started repeating all words and phrases. We were going by the train to Devgarh, a Shiva temple, for my sons' first haircut and Parag started repeating all words on the train. We got so excited and carried away that we bombarded Parag with all the words we could come up with. We knew that this was a big milestone and a pathway for many learning processes. Most of all, he would be able to communicate verbally, which he does now and is able to convey his wants and needs. Every time Parag performed a task or repeated a word or a phrase for us, we would shower him with kisses and hugs. Initially, he was passive and confused by our reactions to his performance. Gradually, he not only started liking being hugged and kissed also responded back. Now he uses these to get his things done by soft hearted souls like grandparents. Actually, Parag loves being with and around people so much that he invades their space and we have to teach him not to do so. I will elaborate on this in the next chapter: Early interventions: Some behaviors we are still working on.

Parag was avoiding eye contact, so this was my next target. I had observed the therapists working with Parag to increase his eye contact. I observed the therapist hold the M&M candy at the bridge of her nose and make a "V" sign with her finger towards her eyes. When he looked at her eyes she would praise him and give him the candy. I started using this strategy with most of his food. I would break a cookie or bread, to increase the frequency of teaching. I also used a pinwheel, for he loved twirling objects. So he followed it with his eyes and I would purposely hold it in front of my eyes, so he made eye contact. This was not paired with food; the wheel was in itself a reinforcer. Giving so much edible stuff for teaching has never appealed to me; it messed up his regular eating routine. Using praise as a reinforcer is very effective in teaching Parag. He loves being praised and it is the easiest way to motivate him to perform. This intervention has worked and Parag looks everyone in the eye.

Parag used to shoot away like an arrow. He did not have a fear of being lost in public places. We had to be so careful when we took him outside. One time we were in the mall and before we knew he had taken off towards the water fountain. I did not want him to get lost, so it was important to train him to be with family. In India my siblings and I took Parag to the park and we would all walk side by side with him. After few days, we all decided to hide behind the trees and shrubs and see what Parag did. He went on walking for a bit but once he realized no one was with him he stopped, looked around and then just stood there looking for us. We came out and he looked relieved to see us. We were very happy to see this reaction because this was the first time he had shown emotion or hesitation and did not walk away without caring. We also taught him to hold hands in crowded places. In 2006, we took him to see the Christmas tree at Rockefeller center in New York. He clutched my hand so tight. The fear of getting lost was in him. Now, he keeps an eye on family members and likes to keep everyone together!

When we go out to movies, restaurants and games, he likes to round us up and make sure that we are all leaving together. There have been times I have forgotten my purse or sunglasses in the restaurant but Parag does not forget. He retrieves them for me. So the fear of getting lost, not only made him keep the family together but he also gained a keen sense of awareness for our material possessions. One time, Parag grabbed a tea kettle at my friend's house and was ready to bring it to our home because we have the same tea kettle. We had to convince him that ours was at home and that this one was not ours. It took almost two years of training till he metamorphosed from Parag the rocket to Parag the herder.

Walking on his tip toes is one of the many symptomatic behaviors. Many children walk on their tip toes, it is a part of the developmental phase they come out of it as they grow. I read that autistic individuals will walk on their toes off and on, even when they mature. I was determined to get rid of as many symptomatic behaviors as soon as possible. I wanted him to blend in well with his normal peers. This helps in social acceptance and this was one of my primary goals. I wanted him to look and behave as normal as possible. So to stop him from walking on his tip toes I bought shoes with a hard sole and made him walk on those. At that time, I was looking for a sabot, since I did not find one I had to settle for a hard, unbendable sole. I made him walk around the neighborhood in them. During this time I also trained him to listen and follow commands like run, walk, and sit down, standup and stop. I would say "Parag let's run" and I would run with him. The same was for walking and stopping, in my neighborhood there was a bench and I would tell Parag "mom is tired, let's sit down" or "mom is rested let's stand up and walk". Also, I made him talk, asking him "what are we doing" and then give him the answer while pairing it with the action. Once he knew words for every action, then I made him expand his answer into a sentence. What I used was **back chaining or forward chaining** of the words. An example of back chaining is when he knew what sitting meant, for he did it when asked and said it too. Then when asked "what are you doing", we would make him repeat 'am sitting' and the next phase was "I am sitting". Once this was drilled he could say the sentence automatically, for he knew this was how to respond to other action words. Forward chaining was easily applied to anything he wanted. We would ask "what do you want" and he would say "I want..." and then he supplemented the thing he wanted, like cookie, coke etc. He knew how to respond and what was expected of him. **A lot of times children with autism are not doing things asked of them, not because they don't want to do it. They don't know how and what to do, for no one has shown them or modeled those tasks for them.** Parag not only stopped walking on his toes but learned many other things that I was able to teach him incidentally, for the opportunity of teaching those was occurring in the context of walking.

There were important skills that he needed to learn that are important for functioning in the society. Potty training was a big thing and I diligently started working on it, when he was three. It was a big milestone in Parag's development. This was the most rigorous training and took me almost one and a half years to get him where he was accident free and was getting up at night and using the restroom. I guess this phase is very challenging for any mother but children with autism take the challenge to another level. The reason for increased intensity for the caregiver who is training is that they have to make sure that this skill is generalized in different settings. It took Parag time to realize that restrooms are available at different places and not just at home. I knew that the potty training was totally internalized by Parag when traveling by car he would say "I want to "potty." I would say "not right now, hold on, we need to find a restroom" and he understood and held on. This was a great achievement for Parag and me as his potty trainer!

This is how I trained him. May be this will help someone else in that ordeal. I would make Parag sit in a chair in front of the restroom with his toys and also give him a good amount of juice and water and after about half an hour I would ask him to "go potty", I wish I had used the word restroom because for it is better to teach words used by an adult, for they grow up fast. We are trying to replace potty for restroom but it is very difficult to undo something taught. It has been hard work but he is now using the word "restroom" also. For bowel movement, I had to be alert about the time he went and make him sit on the toilet a few minutes before. After the deed, I made him look at his creation and made a big deal about it and then made him flush, clean and wash his hands. At night I would wake him up to use the restroom, so that he did not wet the bed. Eventually, he started getting up on his own and using the restroom. The whole ceremonious deal took one and a half years to culminate into perfection. I had to make him realize that bathrooms are available once he expresses his need. While driving on the highway I would ask him, if he needed to potty and if he said "yes", we would take an exit and take him to a restroom at a gas station. After that was teaching "holding on", till he reached the restroom. This was comparatively easy for he got conditioned to using the restroom only when he saw a commode.

In the school he learned to ask permission from the teacher to use the restroom. He has a habit of asking us too. If we are not around and he has an emergency he rushes in. During the training phase I used cotton pull ups which simulates underwear but are padded. If there was an accident then he felt uncomfortable. Getting rid of the regular diaper was a must.

I remember an incident at a rest area. Parag was about four. I took him to the ladies restroom, made him sit on the commode in one restroom stall and then I went to the adjoining one. Well, in few minutes I heard a lady shouting "leave my purse." I rushed out to see that Parag was grabbing the purse from under the slit in the stall and there was a tug of war going between the lady and him. I had stopped breathing. I said loudly to Parag "leave it" and once Parag heard me, he let go of the purse. I grabbed him, apologized to the lady and rushed out. I was so embarrassed and flustered that I did not even wait to face her. When, I put Parag in his car seat I told him, "Parag was a bad boy, keep hands quiet in the restroom, and never touch anyone's purse ever again." Parag knew that he had done something he should not have, for the way I was bombarding him with words of corrections which was a rare thing. After that he was very quiet throughout the drive. I know he understood, for this incident was never repeated again. After that incident I also kept a strict vigil outside his restroom door. Once he was about eight, I let him go to the men's bathroom accompanied by his dad or his brother. We also made him look at the sign in front of the bathroom, which said "men" or "gentlemen." Parag knows that he has to go to the men's' bathroom. When we go to someone's house with Parag, we show him the restroom, so he knows where it is in time of need.

A mother of an autistic kid came to know that Parag was potty trained. She asked me to help her out because he son who was twelve was still not potty trained. I made Parag model for her and then shared my experiences. I also asked her to use the cotton pull ups on her son, so that he should feel uncomfortable in case of an accident. She was too tired by the ordeal and used regular diaper and then was very frustrated that her child was not getting potty trained. **It takes lot of consistent and persistent effort with a tremendous amount of patience.**

Once potty training is nailed down every one's life becomes easier. Particularly the mother's because generally she is the one cleaning up the mess. I have noticed that everyone loves to play with a happy, contended child but the moment the child begins to cry or does potty, he/she is handed back to mother's supervision! Potty training is a great developmental milestone for all children. For a child with autism hygiene and cleanliness is very important for their health and for acceptance in the society.

The next big accomplishment was buckling up in the car. Parag did not like being buckled up in the car and made lot of fuss. While we were in the car, the moment he took off his belt, I would put the flasher on, stop the car re-buckle his seatbelt and then drive again. Looking back I feel I must have been such a driving nuisance those days and I am so thankful for living in a friendly, small town. This was a battle of will power between Parag and me that I knew I was not going to lose. It was essential for his safety that I win. Ultimately, Parag gave in and started to buckle up with the command "put the belt on" and now it is like a reflex action. The first time Parag buckled himself without any prompt, I was elated and my heart sang "hallelujah."

This anecdote is related to putting on a seat belt, in a plane. I was traveling with Parag after his diagnosis. He was three and at that time hated seat belts. The air hostess told me that he had to have his belt on otherwise plane cannot fly. I tried but Parag revolted with fright and might. Flustered I told her that he is autistic and has aversion to being buckled. She was persistent, so I asked her to try herself and when she bent to help Parag, Parag grabbed her hair bun which came rolling out on the side. She got more upset because some passengers laughed. She went to get the pilot, I told him my predicament and he said I could hold Parag in my arms as tight as possible during the takeoff. I am so thankful that he understood and made an accommodation to help. I understand that rules and regulations are very important but during special circumstances a little empathy and an accommodations makes everyone's life easier. It fills my heart that the world is made of understanding and beautiful people.

Parag's training of buckling up is so successful that he not only buckles himself up but will make sure that everyone has done so. Parag sits in the back seat behind the driver's seat and there is no way the driver can drive without the seat belt on. Parag nudges at the driver's back and reminds them to wear the seat belt. The reason he sits at the back is when he was young he had the habit to fiddle with things around him and I was scared that if he sat in the front he would touch the gear or try to play with it. Recently, one of our relatives was visiting us. He sat next to Parag in the car and he did not fasten his seat belt. Parag said to him "belt on" but he did not pay attention to Parag's request. Parag got hold of his seatbelt and handed him the buckle saying "belt on please." I was very pleased to see that my training of making Parag buckle up has extended to where he is making other people do the same. My student has become a teacher in this life skill! These are the moments when I am able to mentally pat myself on the back, pause and enjoy the moment. I feel it is important to pause and enjoy the journey to the successes because they are long.

Teaching Parag the correct use of the word "yes" and "no" was the beginning of the verbal communication. To teach "yes" was easier, for I would ask him if he wanted his favorite toy, or his favorite food, he would extend his hands to get it, at that moment, I would nod my head and would ask him to say "yes". Once he said yes, I would give him what he had shown desire for. "No" was bit tricky. Whenever he did not want to do something, he would start biting his wrist, I would stop that behavior and tell him to say "no" and also make the head gesture for no. For example, reading was something he did not like initially, this was an opportunity to teach "no" because once he said no to reading or to anything else I had to stop, that was the only way he could understand the meaning of the word. So I would say, "No reading now, later". This was to let him know that we will resume this activity after sometime. Long sentences would also confuse him. I had to keep my instructions short. Once "yes" and "no" became clear to him in the context. I started forward chaining, adding words after yes and no. Example- "Yes cookie", after this the next level was, "yes, want cookie" and the "yes, I want cookie." Same with "no", "no reading", next level, "no reading book" and now "no I don't want to read book." Now he realizes he does not have to say "yes" and "no" all the time, he can just say "I want or I don't want". So his communication has variety, he chooses how he wants to communicate, in a word, phrase or a sentence. Teaching "yes" and "no" was a huge stepping stone for communication.

As he learned more vocabulary, he learned to communicate and understand many words that he was hearing all the time. This made him a happier person. Vocabulary is something we emphasize in his curriculum. As he acquires more words with understanding, he is able to communicate better. It automatically improved behaviors, and he is less frustrated. Along with vocabulary, we also taught him sight words (Dolch Sight Words) and phonics. I have written more elaborately about how we taught Parag to communicate in the chapter: Teaching Communication.

Sitting down for formal class work and asking for breaks were also important milestones. It reduced coercion between Parag and the teacher. Parag did not know how to communicate his need to take a break, so he just started biting his wrist or throwing tantrums. To teach Parag the words like "all done", "no more", "finished" "two minutes" and of course "break" has been a life saver. He tells us before he gets too frustrated with tasks. While Parag was performing a task or working on a worksheet, the teacher will say, "take a break." She then asked him to sit in another chair, where he could sit and relax. This was necessary for him to understand that release from work is called a "break." Once he understood this, the teacher started making him say the word "break" before letting him go. Gradually Parag started asking for breaks, when the task became a bit too difficult to handle. Initially, we also paired the breaks with a short activity that Parag liked for example he could flip through his favorite magazine, or listen to one song from his collection, or watch a part of his favorite DVD, or play with his favorite toy. Most of the time, Parag released himself from the task and sat on his couch for a few minutes and then came back to finish his task. If we felt that he was taking more time than he should, we asked him to come to the desk, which he did, if he was ready otherwise he would say "two more minutes." If he did not return to the task then we would say two minute is over, "come now." This was said bit authoritatively and Parag would obey because he knew that he teacher's voice means business. All this required teacher's "withitness". A term which means that a teacher has to have awareness of her classroom at all times and is able to communicate both verbally and nonverbally. **I believe that in teaching Parag, the teacher's ability to perceive before an unwanted event or behavior occurs and her ability to prevent it is a big part of the "withitness."**

He understands dangers like fire and sharp objects, like a knife. I showed him these things along with other sharp objects and would pair the word "ooho." He associated this word with hurt because that is what I said when he fell down or I would ask him to show me the "ooho" and press my hand against his tummy or ear

56

and ask if he was hurting there. I wish I had taught him to say the word "hurt" instead of making this phonetic sound to ask him if he is hurt. When he is hurting somewhere, he takes the caregivers hand and shows where he is hurting and says "ohoo" and sometimes he says the word "hurt" because we are trying to replace the sound "ooho" with the word hurt. All children with autism, including Parag learn through repetition. Understanding pain and hurt can be taught effectively through incidental teaching or through teachable moments.

Parag, like many other kids with autism, had tactile issues. He did not like to touch gooey stuff and dirt. Parag did not like to walk on the grass without shoes on. To desensitize him, I put his toys in a deep tray filled with shaving cream, rice, lentils and sand. Then I asked him to get his toy out. Initially he hesitated but his desire to play with the toys overcame his hesitation to touch the gooey shaving cream or grainy sand. We also made him play with the play dough. We played games on the grass, like running and catching each other. Sometimes there were other kids too. Initially he tried to tiptoe in the grass but running fast was impossible that way, so he gradually started planting his feet on the grass and running. Gardening helped to desensitize him from touching dirt. We started first with plucking fresh vegetables and watering the plants. Once he began enjoying these, I made him plant seeds and plants. We also made him play in the sand box with other kids. All these activities took gradual and gentle immersion. The element of fun overrode Parag's hesitation and aversion to his tactile issues. Parag has overcome his tactile issues because now while making his crafts he has to work with gel, paint, oils, sugar and salt.

It is very easy to overdo teaching. Anywhere I went I would show him stuff and ask him what it was or try to correct his behavior. Looking back, I feel both Parag and I would have been happier if I was a little less demanding. For example, I would go to the Doctor's office, get a magazine and start showing him pictures and asking what it was or a grocery store and start showing him things and ask him what it was. Parag did not like being taught everywhere, so he would resist, most often by biting his wrist. I would try to stop him and all this gave us unwanted attention. After a few altercations, I realized there was a simple answer to all this caco-phony. **There is a place and time for everything and not to put too many goals to an activity.** So, at doctor's office, now my goal is to make him sit quietly. He can take his CD player or I-PAD and listen to it with headphones or he could just enjoy looking at the pictures in the magazine. The goal is for him to sit quietly and properly in the waiting area and in the examination room as well.

In the grocery store, I made him push the buggy and walk along beside me. Basically, he had to behave; this is essential for social acceptance. I wanted him to learn to shop for his grocery, so I set aside a day for that. Before I was getting my groceries and trying to teach him the things he needed to learn at the same time. This was a blunder, for it was an overload of tasks on both the teacher and the student. **The lesson learned was never mix personal work with student's teaching, even when that student is your child!** The moment his grocery day got separated from mine, it became a pleasurable activity for both of us. Initially, I would cut pictures of the stuff he needed to bring from the store, and then I would paste it and write next to it what it was, and make him read it. Parag recognized the picture and knew what to get. He was happy buying his groceries and I would let him buy one item of his choice as a reinforcer for his good behavior. Generally, he chooses chips or coke. Now, the teacher makes him write his own grocery list, he does not need pictures and has a debit card, which he swipes and then signs his name on the receipt. The goal is to not only learn a skill but also to blend in with the people. Parag has to behave appropriately.

Grabbing a teachable moment and contextual teaching are very effective ways to teach early intervention skills. During this phase Parag acquired a functional vocabulary, learned to ride a bike, swim, play Wii, ping pong, air hockey and listen or play music for his own leisure. All these skills have enhanced the quality of his life and ours too. Early intervention made Parag receptive to learning. I have dealt with the issues of other symptomatic behaviors hand flapping, putting hands on the ears, mumbling and biting due to frustration and task avoidance in the following chapter.

Early interventions: some behaviors that is due to sensory input and task avoidance

Children with autism have no control over the behavior that occurs due to sensory input because they don't know how to process it. For example: Tic, hyper extending of the body, flicking their hands, grinding their teeth, mumbling, covering their ears to shut out noises. These are all repetitive behaviors. What adds on to their frustration is their limited language and not being able to express in words. Often this frustration manifests itself as behaviors.

Parag used cover his ears when he encountered a loud noise, like when we used a blender or a vacuum cleaner. We used these around him but for a few minutes and asked him to keep his hands down. Gradually, we increased the time, until these sounds did not bother him. Nowadays he cleans his classroom with the vacuum cleaner and uses the blender for his crafts projects. Parag also resisted listening to music through earphone. When we insisted, he kept it away from his ears, at his temples. Gradually, he started putting the earphone in his ears. The training was the same as with the vacuum cleaner and the blender. We exposed him to the music minimally, when he wore the earphone and slowly increased its time, till it stopped bothering him. Parag loves music, therefore it was easy to persuade him to use earphone. The reason was not only to acclimatize him to listen through an earphone but it is also an appropriate social behavior. It is simple courtesy to the people around and to avoid noise pollution. I also feel that children with autism put their hands on their ears when they perceive that we are talking about them as if they are not present. They know and understand. Putting their hands on the ears when there is no loud noise but just people talking is their way of conveying that they do not like the conversation. I have noticed this in Parag. I have elaborated on this aspect in the chapter "At what level is Parag functioning?"

Parag used to flick his hand and occasionally he still does. Now, he is aware of this gesture and knows that he is not supposed to do it and he tries to control it through the coping skill that we have taught him. When he was young once he started doing it we would say, "hands in the pocket," so he was still doing it but it was not obvious to the people. Moreover, if he had the urge to flick his hand, he would put them in his pocket most of the time. It is very important that he has an outlet for a sensory input. Asking him not to do it does not help. We have to teach him the coping skills and then alternative behaviors. Overtime, the behavior has subsided.

The next thing was to make him understand that he should try to control his hand flicking. We would tell him, "hands quiet, you can control it." To teach him how to control this, we gave him something to hold that he likes. This training started early so at that time we would give him his favorite toy or his favorite book. When he is holding something, then it is physically impossible to flick his hand. If he was sitting down and flicked his hand, we asked him to "put your hands under your legs." All this gave him tools to actively control the behavior, when it occurs.

Another behavior is mumbling. When he mumbles, they are not random words, all jumbled up, but most of the time they are something he has picked from his environment. He used to sing, which sounded like "kue kue everybo kue". It was rhythmic but did not make sense. Then one day I saw him picking up puzzle pieces and saying the same words, I realized what he was saying, he had picked up from Barney episode "Clean up, clean up, everybody cleanup." I was delighted to find out what he was singing and then started working on his pronunciation and enunciation of those words. So many times when we think autistic children are mumbling, actually they are saying words and sentences. Often it is not clear to people. **Imagine how frustrating it would be if we were saying something and no one understood us and they asked us to be quiet. Often this is what happens to autistic individuals.**

When trying to figure out how to help, I have to burrow in to Parag's mind to figure out what is he saying. Mumbling is a behavior that interferes in social acceptance. So first came the coping skill, I made him aware that he was mumbling and asked him to go in the shower, where he can sing and mumble. When he cannot or does not want to control it. So there are times he takes a shower and mumbles away to glory, when he comes out he is calm. Water helps him to calm down as well.

The second step is to come up with an intervention plan. We ask him to actively control his mumbling and give him the reason why. We say, "Parag you cannot mumble, you can control it, Papa, Ankur and Mom do not mumble, you should not either. People love Parag more when he does not mumble. Sometimes we just put our index finger on the lips. He knows he is supposed to control his mumbling and it is funny, for he translates the gesture and says "be quiet." There are times when we ask him to be quiet; he says "no," that means I am not going to control my mumbling and I don't feel like controlling it. When we are teaching and Parag starts mumbling a lot, then we stop the task for a while and start talking to him, so that we can reach out and cancel the internal interference with outside input.

The goal is to make him focus on what we are saying. Using encouragements along with distractions. We begin by saying "Parag is a good boy, he can control his mumbling, let's count to a hundred". We start saying the numbers a little loudly, this makes him listen and then after a while he joins in the counting. We may make him say other things like the alphabet, the name of the months, songs and things he is familiar with that he is able to recite on his own. The point is for him to take over and become distracted from mumbling. Another technique is to let him listen to music on the i-Pad. This makes him focus on the input from outside.

We take Parag to the movies and to the library where everyone is quiet. Immersing him in an environment where there is pin drop silence makes him emulate the same behavior. The caregivers who are accompanying Parag are also very alert to maintain the decorum of the place. Movies at the movie theatre and the books and magazines at the library are distractions/outside input to subdue mumbling. **Immersion is a powerful learning opportunity and it has to be a gradual process.**

It is important for Parag to understand that these behaviors are undesirable and he needs to control them. Before teaching him how to control those, we have to give him coping skills. For example, when someone is drowning, you save them first and then teach them to swim. **The same analogy applies here. Coping skills are like saving the children with autism and intervention plans are like teaching them to swim.**

Many behaviors subside and then come back again. It is like a sleeping or dormant volcano. There are times that these behaviors peak or spike before subsiding. Fortunately if the undesirable behaviors return, we are better prepared to handle them, for we already have repertoire of tested intervention plans! They have worked in the past and they will work again.

Parag bites his wrist when he gets frustrated with some task. This happens in two circumstances. First, he is overwhelmed by the pressure of the work, so he uses it to get out of the work. Second, sometimes he uses biting his hand to get things he wants. We have given in to this behavior when people are around. This has worked for him in the past, so he tests us to see if it will work again. Once we became aware that we are the ones conditioning his behavior we all put out heads together and figured out a plan. The best way to deal with his seeking attention through an inappropriate behavior was to avoid acknowledging those behaviors. For example, if Parag asked for an ice cream and then bit his wrist. We left him after telling him that he cannot get it, because he was biting his wrist. He can have it only when he is not biting for five minutes. Parag did not like being left alone because without the spectators for his tantrums, there was no point in throwing the tantrums or biting his wrist. Once he behaved as asked, he got the ice-cream. Gradually, we increased the time for him to behave a certain way before he got the reward or the thing he was asking for. Thus desirable behavior has increased over time. I have found that Parag displays desirable behavior because he knows that after doing what is asked of him he gets what he wants. Now, he is able to postpone his need for instant gratification once we talk with him. **He listens to us because we listen to him and he also knows we mean what we say.** The behavior of biting for stuff is not eliminated but is rare and we can make him stop by talking. This training is very rigorous in the beginning, but all the hard work and patience pays off. This intervention tests the will power of a teacher and with every successful intervention the teacher proves that where there is a will there is a way.

The first thing is to figure out a coping skill and then an intervention plan to mitigate this behavior. We put a wrist band on to protect his wrist and also give him a hanky to transfer his behavior to it. Biting the handkerchief is an essential coping skill. It always helps me to put myself in Parag's place and analyze. When I am angry or frustrated, I want to vent, so there has to be a way to express feelings amicably, to myself or to others. The handkerchief gives him the means to vent without injuring his wrist. Parag has this self-injurious behavior but he is not aggressive to others.

Parag bites his wrist in the classroom to avoid a task. So we have to see if we can make the task less demanding. The first thing is to reduce the work load. That is, instead of making him finish the entire worksheet, we divide it into two or three manageable parts. Next, pair that work with a powerful reinforcer. "Grandma's rule" works very well, "First eat your vegetables and then you can have dessert". Once Parag knows that if he finishes the tasks he can have a break or his music or a reinforcer that he wants, he is more compliant. Dangling a carrot works most of the time. Third, there is a possibility that Parag's behavior occurs because the skill we are teaching is actually difficult and we need to break it down into simpler steps. That is, fill in the gaps before we can teach that particular skill or task. We have to give him the means to express himself before the behavior. For example, when Parag is frustrated with a task, we have taught him to say "no more" or "I want break." He is expressing his need and it is important to acknowledge it.

Sometimes while I am teaching Parag he tells me "naughty boy." This translates to "I am going to be naughty." The actual translation to me is "I am not going to comply". Now the smart thing for me to do is listen to this warning and strategize. I am extra patient and calm and give him all the reinforcing I can muster. My patience definitely mellows him down. A warning is a great thing for it prepares me for a successful session with him. The amusing thing is he knows that he is not supposed to be naughty but he is going to be anyway. What a rebel! **The point is, these children tell us in words and gestures, but many a times we don't pay heed to it.**

Another behavior that we are working on is to stop Parag from blowing out candles. It was impossible to take him to a candle lit restaurant for he would go to other peoples' tables and blow out their candle. It was embarrassing. He was ruining other people's romantic night out.

This is how we are tackling this behavior. The teacher lights a candle in the classroom. Every time he blows it out, she gives him a reason why he should not do this. The biggest reason is "Parag you can't go to nice restaurant if you blow out candles". Then she lights it back again. When he is downstairs with us we do the same. One day while doing this training downstairs he came to me and said "I want to phoo." Since he did not have the vocabulary "blow out", he communicated to me through the gesture of blowing out the candle, a onomatopoeia! It was funny but at the same time he is trying to express his needs through relevant gestures and phonological sounds/onomatopoeia. This is one of the important features for communication. Now he has the vocabulary and it was deja vu when I heard Parag's teacher saying, "didn't I say no blowing out candle." Parag said, "yes, I want blowing out candle." Parag was letting her know that he is aware of her warning but he wants to do it anyways.

Sometimes getting rid of a behavior is not difficult, for the successful strategy applied in the past, comes in handy. I knew that I needed to put burning candles in his environment so that there were more opportunities to eliminate this behavior. When he was about four, he used to rip apart the audio cassettes and make a pile of the tape. I decided to put the rack of audio cassettes in the living room, on the coffee table, so that it was accessible to him, it was easy for us to monitor his behavior and stop him from ripping the cassette. After a while he stopped. So, I used the same strategy for blowing out the candles. The increased availability of burning candles gave us the opportunity to supervise and stop him from blowing them out. Every time he tries to attempt a behavior that has to be extinguished, we have to give a reason why he should not do it. This makes it an easier and faster process. I see that Parag is able to control his urge to blow out the candles better than before because the frequency of blowing out the candles is going down. The reason he likes to blow out the candle is he likes to watch the smoke and he is mesmerized by it. So the behavior is not extinguished completely. I have a feeling that if we go on with the intervention plan, this behavior will be under control too.

Parag likes to give hugs and kisses to people. We are asking him to limit this only to grandparents, parents and his brother. The hardest part is when he is kissing or hugging our friends and I ask Parag to give them space. They tell me "Parag loves me, why are you telling him to give me space? I don't want space". I explain that he may do it to strangers and they say, "teach him when he does to a stranger". I am happy to see that my friends enjoy Parag's affection. This is a tough behavior to correct because so many emotions are involved.

Parag also tries to invade other people's space by getting too close to them, particularly with people he knows. We are making him stand at an arms distance from us and ask him "give me my space." Also, we are making him stand in a circle if he barges in between two people's conversation. Parag wants to get attention and does not want to be left out, so he tries to step between the two people while they are talking. We tell him to join us and make a circle. He can listen too, and chip in. Parag likes that.

Behaviors can be extinguished effectively with intervention when it occurs. We can create an environment for positive behaviors to occur more often and then try to stop negative behaviors from happening. This is incidental teaching. Planning increases the probability of incident happening. Thus it is true "incidental is not accidental." However, we cannot create a context for all behaviors and teachers have to be alert to situations when the behavior occurs. So some behaviors have to be tackled through teachable moments.

When a certain behavior is recurrent then the whole team has to figure out **why** it is happening. The next step is to figure out **when** and **where** it happens, then everyone has to brainstorm and come up with a **intervention plan** to reduce the behavior and eventually eliminate it. While planning, it is crucial to remember that the student for whom the intervention plan is being charted is a part of the team. The reduction and elimination of those behaviors happen faster when the student takes charge and warns the caregivers and teachers before the behavior occurs.

Parag also tells his caregivers to "be quiet." I am glad that he uses the same tone we have used, that is we have not used it as a scolding but mainly to control his mumbling. He has figured it out that by saying this or saying "leave me alone", people will give him space. I am glad for this because recently, one mother with an autistic child was very upset that her child said "shut up" to her. I knew that this child had just given back what he was getting and not because he was mean. It is very important to teach appropriate language with the right intonations to children with autism.

Another behavior we are still working on is to make Parag aware of appropriate food portions. Parag eats like a glutton, particularly the food he loves. The medicine he takes has a side effect of hunger. He sometimes goes in the kitchen and eats from the pans or pots the food is cooked in. Parag does not rationalize the way we do. I believe all of us are guilty of over eating our favorite food once in a while but we still are able to rationalize and stop most of the time. Parag feels his favorite food is an opportunity to feast and eat till he can finish it . One time I had invited some guests over and cooked meatballs. This happens to be one of Parag's favorite foods. When I opened the container to serve, it was all gone. We had to teach him appropriate food portions. The strategy that we have come up with is to make him ask for food when he is hungry. The next thing after he has asked for food is to have him bring his plate and put the food on the plate for himself and warn him when it is enough.

After trying behavioral intervention strategies for at least three months, we pause and reanalyze to see if it is working or not. If the strategies are not working then we have fine tune it. These strategies need time to be tested. One teacher for Parag who used to come up with great ideas but would never give them time to show results. "Rome was not built in a day." **Behaviors won't be eliminated until and unless it makes sense to the child why or why not he or she should do or not do certain things. It needs time and everyone needs to be on the same page doing the same interventions.**

Also the attitude of the caregiver matters a lot in a behavioral intervention. If the teacher thinks that **a child is a problem**, the most likely method the teacher will choose is punishment. This never works because children with autism are not purposely trying to be difficult. They cannot control certain sensory behaviors until taught or shown how to control them. Thus, the teacher and caregivers have to think that **the child <u>has</u> a problem.** This makes them empathetic. The first step to helping anyone.

Parag's average day

This will enable you to see what Parag does and what skills he is learning. Keep in mind that Parag's school is a dynamic, evolving process that caters to his changing needs. His school starts at 9 in the morning; he is ready to go to his classroom. He has already taken a shower, brushed his teeth and dressed himself with minimum or no direction. On days he does not wake up by eight, I have to wake him up; I am the best alarm clock ever. I say "Parag wake up" and Parag says "two minutes," I say "OK". It is important that he wakes up happy and not cranky and there is no need to pick a battle, which can be avoided by communication. So after a few more minutes, I come back to check on him if he has not gone to the restroom, I say "Parag get up." He tries to test me to see, if he can get away with few more minutes of laziness, he says "Last two minutes". This is when, I am louder and firmer in my tone "No Parag, last two minutes is over, get up". He gets up like a released spring and dashes to the bathroom. **I have reiterated that voice modulation is one of the biggest assets that helps bring compliance and discipline with Parag.** The process of waking up Parag is like a game for both of us. I love the way he peeks from the comforter with only one eye open and then ducks his head under the comforter. The days when I am in a hurry, I put the light on and walk away. He has this compulsion to turn the light off and then he heads to the bathroom. Now we do not have to direct him to get his clothes and clothe himself, he has mastered the skill. In the beginning Parag used to take his clothes to the bathroom from his closet, put them in the basket. On his closet door I had stuck a flashcard on which I have written all the clothes he needed to put in the basket. He read and put the clothes listed there. The list of clothes changed with the season. The regularity of this training started working. Once the teacher rings the door bell, he opens the door. They exchange greetings and then he leads her to the classroom.

There are long term and short term goals, setup for Parag. Instead of an Individualized Education Plan (IEP), we call it a report card. The teacher follows a schedule and checklists the skills and tasks taught throughout the day. She shows Parag what he is going to do throughout the day, so he knows what to expect. Moreover, after finishing a task, she gives him free time or he may ask for it, if the task is making him edgy. She releases him and lets him know what he will be doing next. The daily schedule is written on a white board and is mounted on the wall by his desk.

Before releasing him, the teacher may point to the next thing she is going to teach or ask him "Parag show me what we are going to learn next?" This way Parag knows what to expect and what is lined up for the next sitting. Having a plan takes away confusion and gives structure to the home school. Both Parag and the teacher know what is expected of them. I have a trained professional coming to fine tune the program. When Parag was younger, a consultant in ABA (Applied Behavioral Analysis) came once every month to review the program. Nowadays a retired veteran special education school teacher and a consultant in the Birmingham school system comes to overview the program, as per need. The advantage of having them is that they have imparted objectivity to a school run by a mom. They try to answer our questions regarding, the roadblocks we may be facing in running the program. They bring knowledge from their wider experience, because they deal with and help many special needs students.

After finishing up with the academics (functional math, functional communication), Parag starts doing craft work from 12 to 1:30 in the afternoon. He makes pottery candles, beverage candles, soaps, creams, balms and lotions, magnets. This is a part of his vocational training. Craft work was added from October of 2012.The details about his vocation is elaborated in the chapter: Vocational training. After he is done with crafts, he has to clean up his room, vacuum and straighten up. He has a break for one and a half hours and then his informal school starts. A play buddy comes who plays with Parag like ping pong, air hockey, Wii, basketball, badminton, swimming, bike riding, bowling, skating, going for a walk, exercise. He also goes over some maintenance skills, like flash cards. This way we know that Parag is retaining what has been taught. Parag and his buddy interact for approximately three hours. After that it is Parag's free time in which he listens to music, watches TV with us or just sits around with us. Parag's day is full and never boring. Teaching and learning is happening throughout the day with enthusiasm and fun.

How do we know when Parag is ready to learn a skill?

Some skills are a natural progression from the skills he has learned. Parag shows readiness to learn, by doing something that we have not taught him. For example, he started putting his food in the microwave. He likes his food piping hot. One time he put four chicken nuggets in the microwave for seventy minutes. The whole house started smelling of burnt food and that was how we found out what he had done. I realized he was ready to learn to use the microwave. We had to train him to punch the time so that his food was warm and did not get burnt. We made him put his food in the microwave, made him punch the time for one minute and twenty three seconds. The numbers are horizontally written and in one row. Once the time is up he checks his food and if it needs to go to microwave again, he repeats the process. Popcorn was easy to teach, for all he has to do was put the bag in the microwave and punch the button which says "popcorn". Now we make him read the label. On the readymade lunches he follows the directions. So there has been a progression of the skill. He checks his food and if it is not hot enough, Parag also uses the button on the microwave that says "add a minute."

Parag is ready to cook. I know this because of this incident: he loves fried potatoes called "bhujia" Indian French fries. One day he asked me to cook it, I was so tired and did not want to make it, so I teasingly told him go make it yourself. Later when I went to the kitchen. He welcomed me with a beaming smile. He had put the skillet on the stove, put oil in it and he was frying some potatoes which he found in the fridge. They were already cut. Thankfully, he had forgotten to turn on the stove. Lot of times when I am cooking Parag does his puzzles on the kitchen floor. Often he stands and just watches me cook. I go on talking to him while cooking like, "Look this is onion, mom is going to cut it, onion makes your eyes water." These are teachable moments and over so many years of doing this, grabbing the moment and talking to Parag comes naturally to me. I also make him respond to questions like, "What is this?" "What am I doing?" "What is Parag doing?" I wait for his appropriate response. If he does not give me one then I provide him the answer. Parag's attempt to cook is yet another example that children with autism do learn through observation. He has put clothes from the hamper into the washer. We have to choose what skills we are ready to teach from the things he is showing interest in. Right now, we are teaching him how to make his own bed, taking the dishes out from the dish washer, which he does with gusto for he thinks of it as a game. He also sets the table for dinner. He makes his own sandwich for lunch.

Parag is ready to learn shaving because when we try to help him shave he does not like it. He wants to shave on his own. A few months back I was making him shave hand over hand (he holds his razor and then with my hand on top of his, I guide him to shave). Parag was not happy with the assistance so he took off my hand and started shaving on his own. I was pleasantly surprised and very proud that he is showing signs of independence. We now make him see the spots that he misses. I have described my worries about Parag learning to shave in the chapter: some concerns, issues and future plans. When the time came for him to shave it was no issue at all.

At the same time it is important to know which skill should be taught later, after filling the gap first. Which skill teaching we should stop for it has lost its meaning or has become redundant. We have stopped Parag's music lessons. Parag was rebelling, he showed his resistance in many ways, told the teacher "go away please, no more" then tried to mess up playing the songs that he can play blind folded, for he has memorized them. His last resort was to bite his wrist (we put on a wrist band for this Self Injurious Behavior/SIB).

I decided to stop his sessions for a while because this artistic pursuit was not pleasurable for him. There are many reasons why, he is not enjoying learning music at this point in time. First of all the teacher was making him practice the same songs that he knew and she was not teaching new ones. Parag was bored. I observed many sessions and gave my feedback to the teacher but there was no change in the situation. I realized that the teacher was not motivated anymore. So this part of the program has been discontinued for now.

The bad mood from this carried over into the entire school day causing the classroom teacher to improve his mood and then carry teaching. The important question is: is it worthwhile to carry on an activity that makes him so irritable? To me the answer is "**no**", **until and unless that skill is essential for his life.** Even though the music lessons have been discontinued, he still benefits from it. He has developed a habit of listening to music. He can play songs on the keyboard for fun and pleasure. To be an effective teacher around a special needs child the teacher must possess an ability to perceive the student's mood and interests. Accordingly, the teacher directs the student's attention to the tasks that can be achieved with the least resistance. The important thing is learning and teaching should be a productive and rewarding experience for both the student and the teacher.

Many times parents try to teach or focus their attention on one skill that there child is good at, hoping he/she may be a savant in that field. I feel that a lot of times this takes away the opportunity for kids with autism to become more balanced and well rounded, particularly, when any activity hinders their normal day to day functioning. For example, children with autism can play video games for hours and amazingly well, but they get pretty annoyed when they are asked to stop. Obsession, with or for anything, makes the children with autism show undesirable behaviors and become socially less acceptable.

I believe that the skill they learn should be useful and beneficial to them. They should be able apply these skills for their advantage. If any skill starts to escalate into a behavior problem, then behavioral intervention is required. **Every learned skill has to be used judiciously so that it contributes towards enhancing their quality of life.** All of us want to do more of something that we like, but we are able to switch back to other necessary activities. Children with autism have a very hard time doing so. With proper training and encouragement they are able to switch to activities that they prefer less.

Parag is receptive to learning because his teachers and caregivers make his lessons, skills and tasks interesting for him. They are big on reinforcing. Praises are the biggest motivator for he is so much in love with himself, that praises are his greatest gratification. He works harder if you praise him. His lessons and skill teaching are broken down, so that every mini step makes him successful. We may temporarily discontinue certain lessons and skills because Parag may not be ready to learn that. We have to find a way to fill the gap by scaffolding. For example-When he was four, we tried to teach him our home phone number, which had three sixes in the end and he pronounced the 'i' with an "e" we discontinued it for a while and collected similar sounding words to pronounce .Once he could say those with proper enunciation, we came back to teaching the phone number.

The gist is that Parag's program changes as Parag progresses developmentally and emotionally. This is one of the big reasons that his home school has been moving forward. **In our case, I don't know about slow and steady wins the race, but for sure we are in the race because there is an ongoing progress!**

Smooth sibling relationship and family communication

Once Parag was diagnosed with autism, my attention gravitated towards him and in that process, Ankur my elder son, who is just ten months older than Parag got neglected. I would ask Ankur to go watch TV and that became a means to escape from reality for him. This is the habit he has to still monitor and learn not to procrastinate.

I sent both the brothers to a day care center and Parag was accompanied by a nanny. One day at lunch time a boy grabbed a cookie from Parag's plate and Ankur jumped on that boy, saying "how dare you steal a cookie from my brother." I was there and it took me a lot of effort to detangle both of them. One time the battery of our car died, Ankur who was five then, saw his dad jump start the car with the cables. He came back excited and said "mom I know how to fix Parag's brain." I asked him "how?" He enthusiastically said, "When I will grow up, I will make a special cable, open up Parag's skull and jump start the brain and then Parag will be alright." I laughed and cried at the same time to see so much love and concern Ankur had for his brother. We put Ankur in a private school in kindergarten, once he turned five. After one year we asked the same school to consider having Parag there as well . We wanted Parag to develop social skills and communication through interactions with his peers. The principal and some other staff checked Parag at his daycare to see how he was behaving and how well he was integrated there. One afternoon I had a phone call from the principal that she was sitting with Mr. Mishra and he had convinced her that Parag should be studying in this school. I was totally confused because Pranav was at home, so I said, "but Dr. Mishra is at home." The principal chuckled and said, "Yes but Mr. Mishra is with me" and I realized she was calling Ankur "Mr.

Mishra." Ankur had gone to the principal and presented reasons to the principal for Parag to be in the same school as he. He had many valid reasons, like if Parag was with kids he would stop being like Dopey from Snow-white and start talking. It would be easy for him to keep an eye on his brother. I thanked the principal for her decision but she laughed and said, "You should thank Mr. Mishra." I was thrilled and was so proud of Ankur. He was already showing the signs of an elder protective brother and was being his advocate!

However, over time Ankur must have felt neglected and less loved than his brother. Over the years it built into a silent resentment and pent up anger. When Ankur was in middle school, he started complaining that he could not play and talk to Parag. He said that his friend's brothers and sisters interacted but he was the only one who did not have a normal brother. This made me think that I could take a role of his sister too. I was totally wrong. This made him more confused because the boundaries for sibling relationships are different than that of a parent. I was juggling to be a sibling and a mother. So as a sister, I would kid and joke and as a parent I would enforce discipline. It was a total fiasco and soon both of us realized that, it was better for me to be just a mom! Now, that Ankur is more mature and Parag more interactive and immensely nosy, they have a relationship and bonding which is unique and in my eyes perfect!

One day, when Ankur was in ninth grade, he came back from school, he had fallen and had scraped his knee. He showed it to me and I said "clean it and put on a band aid." That is when his pent up emotions came rolling out. He told me that I did not love him and that I loved Parag. I was shocked and instantly denied his statement. I tried to reason with him and said that Parag is emotionally like a five or six year kid, so I talk to him at that level.

Moreover he is so much in love with himself that I am able to get things done from him by praising him and that Ankur has seen how bad things can go by picking a fight with Parag. Parag gets in the resistance mode. I said that I loved him as much and treated him at his emotional age level. Ankur listened to all this but stood by his statement that I did not love him. So I said "OK, I will prove to you that I love you but you won't like the way I show love to Parag." He looked quizzical but agreed to the challenge.

The next day, I drove him to school, parked the car I got down and started kissing him and saying you are my guju-muju(a word I have made up, more like a baby talk), he turned beet red, embarrassed and looked around to see if anyone was watching us. He said, "MA have you lost your mind, stop." I stopped right then and started laughing. He was still upset, looking at me ferociously, and I said that I had proved my point, that his reaction showed that he did not like the exaggerated expression of love which Parag likes. I told Ankur that I love him as much as Parag for they both are like my eyes and I don't prefer one over the other.

Ankur went to Georgia Tech after high school but in third semester he was put on an academic dismissal for a semester. We found out that he was grasping academically, procrastinating and then escaping into the world of television and new found friends. We were dismayed and it took us time to realize that he needed our support and help too. In high school he did not have to work hard to get good grades but at Georgia Tech that halfhearted effort did not work for him. He was humbled, shaken and lost his confidence. We decided that it would be better for him to acquire study skills and that community college locally was best for him. He got admitted to the community college, which he had not even considered in his dream of dreams and now the same institution came to his rescue. In this college he slowly built himself by learning study skills, a work ethic and the benefits of being consistent and persistent.

I am glad that after coming back home from Georgia tech, Ankur was going to the Community college from home. This gave him and Parag an opportunity to bond with each other in a unique way. This also gave us a chance to enjoy Ankur more, support him better and rebuild communication channels. Now, Ankur is like a protective elder brother and a buddy to Parag. He takes Parag to the movies and to his friends. When Pranav and I go out, we ask Ankur If he can take care of Parag and spend some time with him. If Ankur is free and wants to spend time with his brother, we happily let this happen. Before we did not let Ankur take care of Parag. The main reason was we had read an article about how a sibling of an autistic individual got bitter by taking care of his brother and was very resentful to his parents for making him do so. It was only later in life he came to terms with this. After reading this article both Pranav and I got pensive and decided to not let Ankur babysit Parag or ask him to take care of his brother. We did not want Ankur to feel forced into taking care of his brother. We wanted him to accept his brother and love him too. Looking back I feel this was a radical reaction to an article.

I have started believing, things happen for a reason and we are too myopic to see and understand why. Ankur too has realized that no matter what, his family is always there for him. He is showing signs of blossoming into a beautiful human being with love, compassion, humility and the zeal to succeed. Now, Ankur is going to a college of his choice in Birmingham, Alabama. It is just an hour drive from home so we get to see him on most of the weekends. He chooses to come home and see us.

The family has to adjust and accommodate all nine yards to the needs of a person with autism. Communication is essential for a harmonious family but more so in families who are facing long term illnesses or disorders. Talking and communicating with each other leads to the same frequency and resonance. Ankur had lot of trepidations regarding Parag's future and his own. He feels responsible for Parag in spite of our reiterating that Parag will be taken care of by us and that Ankur is responsible for himself and his own family. This did not calm down his worries, so Ankur and I had a heart to heart talk about how Parag will be taken care of if we are not around. He felt that Parag will live with him and I told him that is not plausible until Ankur's wife and children want that too. Parag is being trained to live in a group home setting, in case of our demise. I told Ankur that he is worried about things which are probability wise fifty years in the future. I told him this only brings worries. We can plan to the best of our abilities but no one knows the future. I also explained that Parag will always need his love and emotional support. I asked him, "what do you recollect about Parag when he was young, how did he behave?" Ankur said that he was totally uncontrollable in every possible way and that his tantrums were never ending. I said "at that time could you visualize Parag the way he is now, happy, totally manageable and actually fun to be around?" He said, "Mom I understand, we cannot change the past and we can't worry about the future that is too far, all we can do is try our best for what we can do with things at hand and first I have to help myself, then I can think about taking care of anyone else". I am happy to see that he is gaining a general perspective about life that will make him strong and not dissipate his energy by worrying about the past or future. I do want him to learn from his mistakes and plan for his future but worrying is an energy dissipater and harbinger of negativity.

When communication stops, it is like flow of water has been stopped. Stagnant water starts stinking. The same happens when there is a communications breakdown. Relationships starts to stink. We talk about Parag because we all deal with the same challenges in helping Parag. Talking and presenting a situation gives a clearer picture and ideas to tackle it. Talking about Parag's challenges has also made us talk about our problems and the challenges that we face individually apart from Parag's. Sometimes the pressure of handling challenges makes us think negatively. It is very important that the family members should pull each other out from this quagmire before it sucks us too deep. **A home that has a person with autism has more emotional ups and downs and camaraderie between the family members is essential.** Parag's autism has brought us closer and it has made us patient, resilient and determined.

Role of Grandparents and friends

I believe Grandparents play a vital role in the growth of their grandchildren and that is why they are "Grand." It took me time to realize how to get the right help from the grandparents. Most of the time they want to help but don't know how, particularly if their grandchild has autism.

In the early phases, when I took Parag to India, my mom turned out to be a big help for me because she is very good at taking care of babies and toddlers. She is a natural, who just enjoys being with young children. This turned out to be a boon for me, because I could let her take care of Parag and could rest knowing that he is in good hands. My dad was more of a counselor and adviser, and a listener. All this was a much needed help then.

Parag's paternal grandparents live in Auburn, Alabama about two hours of drive from our home. This works out perfectly, for they are close by in case we need help. The Grandparents house is a haven, where Parag is free of school and routine. It is a place of fun. Parag knows he can make his grandma do anything for him, by just giving her kisses, hugs and smiles. Parag recites rhymes and slokas (Sanskrit mantras) for his grandpa, which he has taught Parag. This makes grandpa immensely happy and he is very proud of Parag. Just going there and visiting them is a big break for all of us. Parag loves playing hooky from school.

I believe these interactions have worked out for the best of the family. In the beginning when Parag was diagnosed, I wanted all the sets of grandparents to help in the therapy process. I wanted them to teach Parag, so that he can learn various skills. It took me two years to realize that to teach children with autism or any children with special needs is not everyone's cup of tea. It requires training and a heart that enjoys teaching them. Grandparents don't have that specialized training. Moreover they are there to help, not to take over the rearing process of their grandchildren. They have already done their job of raising their children and it is their turn to enjoy the grandchildren. Once I had all this figured out, the journey has been very pleasant. I can relax and enjoy for they are the most beautiful respite, guides and mentors.

Friends play an important role also. They, like grandparents, are also in the dark as how to help. Lot of times they have questions and curiosities as to how we tackle the challenges. We try to answer best of our knowledge and experience. Over the years, I have realized that autism is a mind boggling subject. Every person with autism is different with different sets of challenges in a varying degrees and to top it all there is no cure. So, it is better to keep this conversation as simple as possible and if the purpose of the getting together is to have fun then this is not one of the topics we want to elaborate about. It will soon make everyone's mood very somber.

We love to take Parag to some of our friends house because they have accepted him and love him as he is. It is a blessing to have friends like these. Of course Parag invades their pantry for cookies, chips and ice-cream. During these visits and parties, Parag turns into a caterpillar feeding on all the junk food he can find.

Sometimes my friends try so hard to hide these from Parag but to no avail. I feel Parag has built in radar for junk food because he automatically locates it. One of my friend's had put all the cookies and chips inside the laundry machine, to hide them from Parag. Guess what? Parag found those too. I do not overtly try to train Parag at their house. Firstly, my friends don't like that I try to discipline him at their house. Secondly, I feel everyone needs to splurge and party once in a while. It is better he does it at my friend's house, which means it is an occasional occurrence.

I am thankful to have such friends. They have made our journey of tackling autism, less challenging. Like grandparents, we don't expect them to help us with teaching Parag. The school and people involved there are responsible for that. They know what to do and also how to do it. Friends and grandparents can become an active participants in the teaching process of the child with autism. Then the dynamics changes, it requires scheduled time commitment. They also have to learn how to teach without behavioral melt downs from the child with autism. I wanted grandparents and friends to love and spoil Parag. Give all of us a break from the routine and be a blissful respite and support!

At what level is Parag functioning?

Emotionally, behaviorally and cognitively, Parag is at different levels, so it is very hard to say he functions at a particular age level. I think that if I describe some of the things he does, it will help the readers to figure out for themselves. I have already talked about the behaviors and behavioral interventions in chapters thirteen and fourteen. In this chapter I will write about emotional and cognitive responses .

Emotionally- If Parag sees us dressed up, he knows we are going out. He goes in his room and comes back wearing nice pants and shirt, this is his way to express, "hey, take me with you." Parag knows that to go outside he has to dress differently. If he realizes that we are not going to take him with us, Parag keeps a tight vigil on us. We tell him that we have to go to an appointment or a dinner without him and that we will always come back to him. In spite of all this talking he does not want us to leave him at home. We have to sneak away. Once he realizes we are not there he is fine with the baby sitter. When we come back, he sometimes says "car ride", which means "I want to go out too". There are times we give him a car ride and sometimes when we are tired we just tell him that "we will do that tomorrow". Recently, my husband and I had planned to see a movie in the movie theatre. Parag saw us and realized we were ready to head out. He went to his room, dressed up and came out fast to accompany us. We could not help laughing at his alacrity! We took him to the movies with us!

He does not like to say "bye" to family members for it means that person is leaving him. Parag sees me picking up my purse and car keys and he latches on to me like crazy glue. This behavior is improving now, as long as one of us is at home, he lets the other person go and says "bye" to the person who is going. He likes to keep the family together. He will not leave any of the family members behind in a restaurant, movies, or a friend's house; he rounds everybody up before leaving. Parag is aware of his surroundings. He scans the place to see if there is anything of his interest. For example, last year when we took him to the "Dragon Boat Race" a competition of racing boats in the Coosa river in our town. Parag asked for a coke. I looked around and did not see any so I said "go get it." Parag took off to a booth where people had stacked sodas. Once I knew his intentions, I had to stop him and then take him to a vending machine. It was a teachable moment for both of us. The self-help skill "go get it." works at home but in public I have to be careful. For Parag the learning was that he cannot have other people's sodas, he can have it from a vending machine.

Parag is very possessive of people he loves. When he was young he did not show any attachment to people or things except for the things that increased his self-stimulatory behaviors, like twirling things and small cars that he loved to line up. When Ankur went to Georgia Tech, Parag started sleeping in his room, his way to show that he was missing his brother. One time when Ankur left for college and Parag realized that Ankur was not at home he started crying so much that we had to call Ankur on the phone and make him talk to Parag. This consoled Parag. So Parag is emotional and loves everyone and wants to be loved.

Now when he sees my husband and I are holding hands, he will get in between us and hold our hands. One time Pranav and I were taking a stroll outside our house in the drive way. Parag saw us and locked us out. When we rang the doorbell, he stood there watching us through the glass paneled doors with his hands on the hips. A gesture to show us he was upset at us for not including him. He makes sure that he gets hugged and kissed as well. Parag does show jealousy and competes with Ankur for affection. If Parag sees Ankur lying on the bed next to me, watching television, he will ask Ankur to "go away." Parag tries to pull off Ankur and when Ankur gets off the bed, Parag will immediately take his space.

Parag is also possessive of his favorite things, but in a healthy way. Recently, I bought sandals for both the brothers. I realized the strap of the sandal was rubbing at Parag's heel, where he had a bruise. So, I bought him two new ones without the straps and asked Ankur to use Parag's sandals with the strap. Parag saw Ankur wearing his sandals. Parag did not like that so he went to his brother and pointing at the sandal says "sandals." Ankur asked "what do you want?" Parag said "give me sandals," he stood his ground till Ankur gave him back his sandals and Parag put them on right away! We all were tickled by his possessiveness and determination to get back what belongs to him! Kids with autism show possessiveness to things with which they perseverate or stuff that leads to self-stimulatory behaviors, such as lining up objects or rotating objects. If it is taken away from them they throw big tantrums. This kind of possessiveness is not healthy because it interferes with their normal development. Parag is showing a sense of ownership over his things and we all like to guard what is ours. That I believe is the norm!

If he sees us sitting and talking or watching a show, he comes to check if we are doing something fun without him and if he thinks it is fun stuff, he just joins in. Parag loves the TV show "Jeopardy" and if we flip the channel, he will say "no" and if we don't flip it back to the channel, he will take the remote flip it back and then make sure that the remote is out of our reach but within his reach.

On Valentines day, I make Parag give flowers and candies to some special friends for their support and love for Parag and our family. Last year Parag went around giving those, when he came to the last friend, he gave her the flowers but was not willing to part with the box of chocolates. My friend and I laughed. Parag was looking at us and trying to understand why it was funny. For him it was serious, this was the last box of chocolates and he wanted it for himself. I made him give it to her anyway, in spite of her protests that Parag could keep it. He needed to learn the socially appropriate behavior that gifts are for giving.

A common misconception is that children with autism do not show feelings. This is not true. Parag shows emotions and so do other children with autism. They show emotions and are also aware of their feelings, the only limitation they have is they don't know how to express them in a proper social way. **Actually, behaviors are outbursts of some thoughts and feelings that they don't know how to express in words.** Many children with autism, put their hands on their ears when they hear loud sounds, like a blender or vacuum cleaner. The loud noises and sounds seem to bother them and they try to block these sensory inputs by putting their hands on their ears. I feel that they also cover their ears because many a times we talk about them as if they don't understand. Even worse is when we talk as if they are not present. **I think they also cover their ears, to express their feelings, it is sometimes a gesture to convey that they do not like being talked about.** Parag no longer covers his ears when he hears sounds of the blender or the vacuum cleaner, due to gradual exposure and acclimatization of these sounds. He covers his ears when he hears us talking about him. It is his way to express that he does not like to be talked about. He likes to be involved in the conversation. Parag loves being addressed and making direct communications. Often he just sits and listens to all of us talking. If he feels that we are ignoring him then he directs our attention to himself by asking us for something. It is amusing; sometimes Parag starts to cough when he does not get attention. This is a learned behavior, when Parag coughed, I used to make a big deal about it and give him lot of TLC (tender loving care). Now when Parag feels he is being neglected in a group setting, he starts fake coughing to seek my attention! Parag loves people who acknowledge him and interact with him. He goes to them and initiates communication by giving them hugs and smiles. He sometimes call them "honey mui" this is his special word that he has coined for special people in his life. He listens to me talk in Spanish and I think he has picked this word "mui" from me, which means "very". However, I don't know why he has paired honey and mui together. Maybe he is trying to tell his special friends that they are very sweet. **Who thinks that children with autism cannot communicate? They do, but do we see and listen?**

Parag is very intelligent and perceives heated discussions. He connotes loud tones of voice to unpleasant interactions and he tries to stop it too. When Pranav and I start talking loud he puts his hand on our mouths, a gesture which conveys "please don't talk loud, I don't like it." All he says is "be quiet". Parag does not like to be called "baby." The moment you say that he will correct you and say "no, big kid." There are many TV commercials that emphasize children saying they are big. For example, the Huggies pull-ups, the kid uses the bathroom and says "I am a big kid now." I assume that television commercials like these and our praising him for doing a task independently, Parag has associated that being a big kid is praise worthy and so that is what he wants to be.

Parag is curious and curiosity is the first step towards learning and being aware of the environment. When I come back after shopping, he looks into the shopping bag to see if there is anything that he may like. If I tell him that the shirt is for him, he is happy and sometimes he wants to try it right away. Talk about instant gratification! The same goes for my grocery shopping. He will peek into each bag to see if there is something of his interest and liking. If there is he will ask for it. Parag loves to open the Christmas gifts. It is a sheer pleasure to see him so happy opening the gifts. This year he opened his gift boxes, he was so thrilled to get a red jacket and pants which he wore right away. He loves to go shopping and enjoys trying on clothes. He also carries his own shopping bags. Once we are home he will wear his most favorite one.

Parag is very protective. When he perceives danger he tries to protect himself and the people who are with him. For example- When we went to the aquarium at Atlanta, he was elated to watch the marine animals. In the aquarium they let the people touch the sting rays. When I asked Parag to touch them, he refused. when I tried to do so, he pulled my hand away saying "no." I asked him "Why?" He said "ohoo" the onomatopoeia he expresses for pain. I asked Parag, "do you think fish will bite me?" Parag said, " yes bite." I really wonder why some literature on autism says that the kids with autism don't show emotions and that they don't care.

Sometimes children with autism are a handful to manage at public places, so parents and caregivers avoid taking them out or decrease the frequency of their outings. Social behaviors can be learned better with exposure to the real environment and through contextual teaching. Parag was a handful too, but we chose to take him out to shops, malls, libraries, friends' houses and parties. This way he got plenty of interaction with a variety of people and we got a lot of opportunities to teach him social cues and appropriate social behaviors. In the beginning we used exaggerated body language, voice modulations with facial expressions. Once he understood the emotions, we toned those down because over time he was aware of the subtleties of these social cues. **We made sure that if we used command language with Parag then we also gave him reasons why he could or could not behave in certain way or he can or cannot do certain things. This is so important because children with autism understand. I have observed that rarely people try to explain things to the children with autism; the interaction is command language without any explanation. No wonder they develop a mechanical personality because mechanical responses are what they are being trained for. Emotions come when we talk, not when we give instructions and commands!**

Cognitively- He understands receptively way more than he can express in words. For example- recently I asked him where was his buddy, he went and got her by the hand and brought her to me. He did not ask her verbally. He follows multiple commands around the house. For example, when we ask him to get ready, he goes to his room, gets dressed and comes back to us. When we ask, he puts the lights off and also closes the doors. Parag's biggest limitation is expressive language. We are working on this and I have elaborately written how we are trying to increase his expressive communication skills in the chapter: Teaching communications. He expresses his wants and needs in his limited vocabulary. Increasing his vocabulary is still one of the important teaching targets. Once he has the words to express himself he remembers them and he is also able to generalize them .

Recently, in the car Parag looked at me and said "P." He repeated it and I was not able to understand what he was trying to express. So I said "show me" and he pointed his finger to the dash board and showed me the symbol "p" for Pandora. He was asking me to put the music on Pandora. He listens to music through Pandora, on his i-Pad and also on his teacher's phone, as a reward for performing a task. When he saw the symbol in the car, he knew he could listen to the music also through his favorite channel in the car and he was asking me to put on the music. This is generalization or spillover. It also shows that Parag is trying to communicate his needs and wants. This incident also taught me that now I have to teach him to say "Pandora." As I have said before lots of teaching gets incorporated by incidents and interactions! What separates him from regular people is that he cannot lie. For example- When there is a task he does not want to do, he will say he wants to potty and if you ask him "Parag do you really have to go potty," then he says "no". It is amusing to see such innocence.

Parag is a biological GPS. He remembers roads by the restaurants and gas stations. In the evening Pranav gives us a short cruise in his car, in town. The moment he backs the car from the garage, Parag demands "chips". What he is conveying to his dad is that he wants chips from the gas station at the corner of the road. Pranav buys chips for Parag from that gas station. He remembers every gas station, where we have bought chips for him because all we have to do is drive on the road where the gas station is and Parag will say chips even before that gas station is visible. The next thing he will say is "hungry, French fries" because he knows McDonalds is ahead. As Pranav drives further and crosses the bridge, Parag says "ice cream" because Dairy Queen is on that road. Parag says "Pizza" once we are driving in Rainbow City, for he knows that is the way to Pizza hut. When we go to Atlanta, once we are on I-20, he says "lucche," an Indian snack. He knows that he gets in an Indian store in Atlanta. What is surprising and fascinating is he mentions all his favorite food before he has even arrived there. **He just remembers**. Also, if we don't give him anything he is not distraught or throws a tantrum, he goes on reiterating. He has tested the power of reiterating his demands and he knows that we have succumbed to this pressure. Parag is intelligent and from his experience he knows that history repeats itself and by reiterating his demands he has a better chance of succeeding. Parag is happy to get at least one thing, generally it is chips and occasionally it is ice-cream during the car ride. What the readers need to know is that he does this more when his dad is driving the car because by mentioning these foods, he has been able to get them from his dad. When Parag is with me or Ankur, he does not display this habit because we have not entertained his demands. Parag is not only a GPS for Fast food restaurants and Gas stations but also intelligent enough to know who will give him the stuff he is asking for. This is not simply cognition, that is, "thinking" but this is metacognition "thinking about thinking." **Simply put, it means using your knowledge and experiences for your own benefit and survival.** Parag displays this in abundance in a variety of contexts.

Problem solving is an important aspect towards independence. Parag tries to figure out a lot of thing on his own. There are times it works for him and there are times it does not. The important thing is he is trying to find solutions to his problems or ones he thinks are problems. For example- one time his helium balloon went up to the ceiling, he got a chair and stood on it to grab it but finding it unreachable, he went to the laundry room got a broom, stood on the chair with broom in his hand to reach it. I was tickled to see him think for himself and he looked so cute trying to figure out his problem.

I remember Parag must have been four; he was jumping on the trampoline in the backyard. I went in the house for something and when I came out, Parag was jumping naked on the trampoline. I shouted, "Parag put your clothes back". He was laughing and trying to jump high. He pointed at the neighbor's pool and said "swim." I realized he was jumping high, so that he could catapult himself in the neighbor's swimming pool. He did not care if he had swimming trunks on; skinny dipping was all right with him. I understood his intentions and I laughed my guts out.

Another incident was when all his videos got erased in his i-Pad. He tried to charge it at his regular spot but when that did not work, and he unplugged it and put it at other socket. Even though that was not the right solution, but he was thinking on his own as how to fix the problem. After trying and finding out that his strategy did not work, he gave the i-Pad to me. I was amused and asked him "what do you want?" He said "help". The next thing is make him say it in a sentence, which he does, once reminded. Recently, he brought one of his audio books to me, along with a screw driver. The reason was that the audio was not working because the batteries were dead. He has seen me change the batteries before by using a screw driver to open the battery compartment. So from the past observation, he realized it was time for batteries to be changed and came to me with the right tool. I was delighted and used this opportunity to further enhance the learning process by helping him use the screwdriver to open the battery compartment and put the batteries in. Parag is trying to problem solve on his own and then if he is not successful, he asks for help. This is a life skill, trying to solve problems on our own and when we are not able to then we approach someone from whom we expect the solution.

Parag has uncontrollable sweet tooth and gusto for junk food like chips and cheese puffs. He eats raisins, dates and fruits which are healthier choices, which I have tried to put in his diet. He likes these too but he does not rationalize like we do and try to avoid unhealthy foods. He eats totally for gastronomical reasons; he prefers to eat food that tastes better to him. He is a born Epicurean. The fact that he overeats is also because of the medicine he takes, to control some of his symptomatic behaviors. One of the side effects of this medicine is hunger! I have a lock on my pantry to stop Parag from invading it. The locked doors also give him the increased opportunities to verbalize his demands. I hide the pantry key, he tries to find it. In the movie Jurassic Park, the dinosaurs used to check the fence for weaknesses in the same way Parag gauges the possibilities of my weaknesses as to where I could have hidden the key. There are times he finds it and then he will hide it at a different place. If I ask for it he laughs and will say "no." If I threaten him, he laughs for he knows my threats are empty. I have to plead quite a bit before Parag shows me the hiding spot. It is like a game between us and Parag loves to outwit me. I have to humbly accept.

Once Parag got burned by hot water from the faucet. Since then he uses only cold water to wash his hands and if he sees other people using hot water he puts off the faucet and starts cold water for them. As I have described before he is protective towards others as well. However, in the shower he sets the faucet to warm and then takes a shower. He must have realized taking shower in cold water is not fun. **One thing about teaching problem solving is that the child has to first see the problem.** The teacher was teaching Parag to vacuum his classroom. That is one of his chores to do, once he is done with formal teaching. However, he was not vacuuming well. His teacher and I talked about this and realized the reason he is not performing his task as expected is he is not seeing the reason why. The teacher spread small bits of paper all over the rug and once Parag saw those, he was working hard to vacuum them off. Parag could not see dirt in the rug, so vacuuming was meaningless to him. Parag like any student, needs to see a purpose to learn and perform a task or a skill. Gradually, the teacher is reducing the bits of paper on the rug and then it will be totally eliminated. The lesson learned as a teacher is that if we want our students to become good at problem solving, the first thing is to make them see the problem and then give them tools and means to solve. Gradually take away the prompts and cues. **An educator gets into the student's mind and then tries to solve the problem at their level. If the problem is solved and is way beyond the student's cognitive level, it still remains a problem because they cannot comprehend it or use it for their benefit.**

There are lot of books and papers on autism saying that children or individuals with autism lack emotions. Thanks to the iconic movies like "Rain man," generating this mass image of people with autism, which shows them as computer or mathematic nerds but socially inept. I believe this happens when a child with autism does not receive social interactions and social interventions. Parag was not curious when he was young, he would sit in the corner; play/perseverate with his toys for hours. I believe the early intervention and exposure to people and involving him with the activities that we were doing made him interactive or should I say overtly nosy! I love the fact that he is curious, seeks attention and shows emotions and affections! I am glad that Parag is thinking for himself. He tries to figure things out. A lot of his ideas don't work for him but neither do mine. The amazing thing is he goes on trying.

Behavioral interventions that have worked for Parag

After so many years of behavioral interventions, it is easy to take Parag to restaurants, movies, games and on trips. Sometimes, an eliminated behavior may manifest itself again. These behaviors are like dormant volcanoes. They may erupt all of a sudden one fine day. Behaviors that have been extinguished in the past are comparatively easy to deal with, for strategies to eliminate these are already in our repertoire from past experiences. In this chapter I have elaborated extinguishing of some negative behaviors through anecdotes. I believe this enables the readers to visualize and relate better.

I want to relate a behavior that occurred during shopping at Wal-Mart about two years ago and how I was able to extinguish it. Wednesday is Parag's day out in the community. He goes out with his teacher, to do his grocery shopping and anything else they have planned to do that day, like going to the library or going to the museum. The day before they discuss (verbally and in writing) what they will do on Wednesday. One time in Wal-Mart he threw a fit to get the book Thomas The Train; the teacher was hesitant to buy the book for it was $20 and buying it meant encouraging this behavior. She called me to ask what she should do. I asked her to buy it and take it away from him in the car. This was the easiest way to avoid bad behavior and a tantrum at a public place. I also asked her to let him know that he has been a bad boy. I asked her to take Parag to Wal-Mart every Wednesday, sit in the car in the parking lot and remind him that he was a bad boy in there, so he can't go in. After about a month, I asked her to test and see if he would behave and buy only the things that were on his list. She asked him if he was going to be a good boy inside the Wal-Mart, and when he said "yes", she took him inside and he was well-behaved. The intervention plan worked!

Now that Parag has matured, my strategy to correct his behavior is different than when he was younger. When he was little, it was easy to just take him in my arms while he was yelling and crying and put him in the car and then let him know that he has been a bad boy. Ultimately, he realized that the car was my terrain and I could sustain all his tantrums in there, I would not budge until he quit his tantrums. I figured out that soon Parag would be too big to just pick up and put him in the car when he was creating a public scene. I started teaching him that if he behaved well and did not touch things in the shop except the ones that were on his list, then he could have one treat. Generally it is coke or a bag of chips. This strategy has been a life saver. Now, many times he does not want a treat. Going out is a change from the routine and he eagerly waits for his Wednesday: the day out in the community.

About three years ago, Parag started putting a whole roll of toilet paper in the commode and then flushing it. Water overflowed and it was a big mess. I decided to make him clean his own mess. All the while telling him, if he puts the whole roll of toilet paper in the pot, he will have to do the cleaning. I made him put on the gloves and take out all the soggy toilet paper from the toilet first and then mop the floor. He hated the chore so much that this behavior vanished in no time. **Lesson learned: if you make a mess, you will clean it too.**

There was a time when Parag used to throw his spoon in the trashcan after eating. I found that my spoon rack was looking sparse and when I checked the trash can, I found a couple of spoons there. Like Archimedes I had my "eureka" moment. Parag was throwing a plastic spoon in the trash in school after eating lunch. He was doing the same at home only the difference was this was silverware. I had to show him to discriminate between the plastic spoon and a silverware spoon. This method of teaching has a technical name **"discrimination learning."** In a layman's term it is a method of teaching where the student learns that things are similar but not the same. For example, dogs can be a Pomeranian, a Labrador or a Saint Bernard. They are similar because they are dogs (category) but they are not the same. They vary in shape, size, and looks. The same concept went with the spoon, both the plastic spoon and the metal spoon are spoons but they are still different.

At home I started giving him a plastic spoon to eat with and then ask him to throw that in the trash can, telling him that we throw these in the trashcan after eating. When he ate with the metal spoon, he had to put that in the sink. I let him know that the metal spoon is reused. I also asked him to show me which one was a plastic spoon and which one is a metal spoon. Once he discriminated between the two, the next question was show me which one we throw in the trashcan after eating and which one we put in the sink after eating. After persistent teaching for a month, Parag nailed it down. Generalization has not been an issue with Parag, once he learns something; he remembers and generalizes on his own. So once we teach him a skill, he applies it in different places and surroundings successfully.

Parag used to pinch people, when he did not want to perform a task. The intervention plan was simple, if he pinches you; you pinch him back and tell him not to do it because it hurts. This worked because he did not like to be pinched back. The teacher would perceive that he was about to pinch her and she would warn him before the behavior occurred. This made Parag stop. Don't connect this intervention to punishment because I believe punishment is futile. I felt he needed to know how it feels to the other person when he pinches them. He needed to gain a simple understanding that he does not like being pinched because it hurts. This is exactly how people feel when he pinches them.

I believe that behaviors that are aggressive to others make the children with autism less acceptable. Actually, anyone with aggressive behaviors towards others would be less acceptable. One of the most important goals is to make Parag socially acceptable and for this goal to be successful, he cannot display aggression to others. All behaviors need to be tackled early on but aggression to others needs to be strictly dealt with. The reason is, as they grow older these behaviors increase in frequency and force. When children with autism reach puberty, with testosterone levels going high in the boys, these behaviors can turn into nightmares. This situation would never happen if active persistent and consistent efforts are taken by the caregivers early on to mitigate and eventually eliminate these behaviors. "A stitch in time saves nine."

During the initial phases of home school Parag used to run away from the classroom. He looked for an opportune moment when I was lacking "withitness" and he bolted. Teachers need to have coping skills too, just like the special needs students. The first thing I did was to get locks put on the classroom doors and lock them. So if he left his desk and stood by the door because he did not want to do the task or just did not want to be in the classroom, then he had to say that. So by making this change, I had created a situation for him to talk and convey his need verbally. This was a practical approach and an opportunity for teaching him incidentally. I also told him that he can do the work downstairs at the kitchen table. If he wanted to be away from the classroom that was fine with me but he still had to complete his work. In homeschool, even though I believe it is important to create a place for school work; teaching can happen anywhere in the home. Once he realized that he would not be able to escape work by getting out of the classroom, he stopped running out of the classroom.

Sometimes when I have company, problems with homeschooling can arise. Parag is distracted and wants to visit with my guest. Particularly, when he can hear us laughing and talking. He wants to join the fun too! We sometimes let him join us. I know this is against behavioral conditioning principles but real life situations need learning beyond behavioral conditioning. Parag has autism and children with autism shy away from social interactions and gatherings. Including Parag with our guests is a social learning opportunity for him. I am happy that Parag is not a recluse but he has become gregarious!

In training Parag for various behavioral interventions, I have come up with plans that work in most cases. It just needs tweaking here and there and customization is possible for target behavior. **It has taken me time to figure out which behavior can be extinguished by not paying attention and which ones need enthusiastic approval and reinforcements.** For example, when he used to pitch a tantrum to get out of a task, he would come to my face yelling and crying, and that was the time to say nothing, no eye contact, basically give no reaction. The very reason he was yelling at my face was to get a reaction. To master not to show any reaction has been a challenge, but a worthwhile one. It communicates without words, who is in charge. It is challenging because every such interaction becomes a war of will, whoever gives in first loses. It is important to keep in mind that while teaching, the teachers have to pick and choose the battles they want to win. **It is better to lose some battles when our goal is to win the war.** Reinforcing Parag for performing a skill or an appropriate behavior is a piece of cake. Parag loves being praised and being enthusiastically vocal helps in these situations. Everyone likes a pat on the back for a job well done and Parag is no different. This is a pleasant interaction, where both the parties feel successful.

I want the readers to know that these behavioral interventions have worked because they were used consistently and persistently, when they occurred until the behaviors were eliminated. Behavioral interventions need time and the team has to be on the same page. Everyone follows the same protocol.

Teaching Communication

I have briefly touched this topic in the chapter "Early interventions: Teaching life skills. I feel that elaboration of teaching communication may come in handy to some parents and teachers. Also, one gets to visualize the intensity. Enhancing and acquiring communication skills are rigorous and an ongoing process in Parag's case.

There are various strategies that we employ to increase Parag's communication skills. The three major deficit areas that the children with autism have are communication, social skills and behaviors. Now that behavior is not an issue and largely under control due to various behavioral intervention strategies, we mostly work to increase Parag's communication. Increasing communication reduces Parag's frustrations of being ignored and not being understood. This reduces his asocial behaviors and by default he becomes more social. Of course, we have taught him things like shaking hands, waving bye and replying to overtures like: "How are you?" He says "fine thank you" and we find teachable moments to use words like: please, sorry and excuse me. We give him time to say these on his own, if he does not, we remind him.

The school system emphasizes on fluency of reading accurately and quickly. They believe that fluency leads to comprehension. This approach may be true for children who don't have learning disabilities. We are teaching Parag to communicate by using words and sentences with comprehension, which is more important than fluency. The school system is not working in terms of enhancing communication skills, they are thinking in terms towards making every one into an avid reader. First "learn to read" and then "read to learn."

In 2000, a mother of an autistic child invited me to observe her son, for he was reading fluently but with little comprehension. I observed that he was reading fast and with appropriate diction. When the therapist started asking him questions from what he had read, he did not know the answers to any of those questions. During my internship for my Masters degree, I came across another student with a learning disability he could read but could not comprehend. I started working one on one with him. I applied the teaching suggestions and methods, I had made for the child with autism I had observed before. These teaching methods I was already incorporating with Parag and he was responding positively to these skill trainings.

The first thing I did was to make flashcards of those words from the paragraph. I checked to determine if he could read those clearly and understood the meaning also. If he did not know those then we worked on those words. We tried to understand the meaning of the words through picture flash cards and showing the real object that we were talking about. After telling the student the title of the story and what it was about, I started **chorus reading** (both of us reading together) with my student. This made him slow down and pause at the right places. What I had noticed in both the children was that they read in a monotone without pausing. I made him stop after reading every paragraph, asked him questions, mainly **"what"** questions, the answers to which were obvious and in the paragraph. In the beginning, I made him read or look at the picture where the answer was and repeat it to me; gradually I waited to see if he would try to find the answer on his own. Once he mastered that, we went on to **alternate reading** (He had to imitate my pace after I read, which was slow but loud and clear).Slowing the pace and then asking questions, what, where, which, when, how and last of all why. When the student started answering the **why** questions,

I knew he had arrived, he could guess answers from in between the lines! Of course, with every small success he made, I rewarded him with edible reinforcers, pairing it with praises, until he too like Parag, became hooked on to praises and worked hard to get them, he worked harder. In three months and fifty minutes of this training for five days a week, he improved with leaps and bounds.

After my experiences with both these children, I made a promise that Parag would comprehend whatever he says. He would communicate meaningfully and whatever he reads he would understand. Parag's school differs from a regular school because we emphasize comprehension, and then fluency. Making promises are easy but to follow through is hard. I knew to keep this promise to myself, I needed a plan. First I had to figure out where to start and what problems Parag was facing while communicating. He was having a hard time pronouncing "r", "l" and "s" sounds. We started working on the letters that he was having problems with. We got a lot of work sheets for him to work on these letters and we made him slow down and listen to us. We emphasized the letter sound he was having trouble with and then made him say the word. For example he said "poon" instead of "spoon", so we made an elongated "s" sound. This stretching of the letter sound made him imitate better and pronounce more accurately.

To communicate he needed to learn sight words, these are the most frequently used words in the English language. It is called a sight word because it needs to be recognized by sight that is, memorized because a lot of them cannot be sounded out. You may ask, well aren't these prerequisites for fluency? The answer is yes but these are a vital requirement for communication and we were not working on "quick reading" but correct pronunciation and enunciation and the acquiring of words (sight words). The research says fifty to seventy percent of any general text is made of sight words. To communicate, acquisition of these words is essential. Along with this we were teaching Parag to sound out letters of the alphabet, which if I wanted to make it fancy I would say we were teaching him to phonetically decode words.

We also started teaching him action words and making him do those actions as well. We would write the action words on a flashcard, ask him to read it and then model the action. He had to imitate those. To check if he got it, we asked "show **jumping**," and if he performed the task correctly every time, it was time to extend it. We would write Parag can jump; each word on a separate flash card. His task was to listen carefully and put those cards in the right order. The sentence got longer as he realized what was being asked of him. For example: Parag can jump high. Parag can jump high on the trampoline. Parag and Ankur can jump high on the trampoline.

As he went on acquiring sight words, we began to use sight word readers. Since our goal has been comprehension, we asked him questions by making him look at the pictures emphasizing on a target word more, for example "jump." First we made him touch the pictures like "touch boy, touch cat". What is the cat doing? We wait for an answer. If he did not answer, we made him read the portion with the answer again and then ask again "What is the cat doing?". If he answered then we praised him. If he did not we said look, it says "the cat jumps", we point at the word **jump**. Once Parag answered, we extended it to: can you show me jumping, once he jumped, we extended to: where Parag jumps, giving him the answer, "Parag jumps on the trampoline". After a couple of practices we asked the question and waited for his answer. If he answered we praised him, if he stumbled; we prompted him towards the right answer. Eventually he was able to answer without any prompts. We sometimes asked: do you want to jump on the trampoline? If he said yes, we took him to jump on the trampoline, and while he was jumping, we asked what is Parag doing and made sure he answered: "jumping" and once this verb made complete sense, we made him extend the answer to "I am jumping" and then "I am jumping on the trampoline". This is **contextual teaching** and is very important for comprehension and for generalization. This solidifies the concept in a concrete way. The extensions are immense. For example, if I too jump, then I say "mom and Parag are jumping" and then extend it to "we are jumping." "We two are jumping". If Ankur joined us "Ankur, Parag, mom are jumping, we three are jumping." This way we also introduced numbers, but in a more meaningful way. We also make him work on the computer, with discreet trial training, he had to differentiate between walking, jumping, running etc. The same concept is reiterated visually, asking him to click on a particular action word. We got another story which had word jump in it, because reading the same story again and again becomes boring. For example "The red sock jumps" before we read the story, we worked on new vocabulary words. This story adds concepts of color, a good way to review those. We made him watch Winnie the Pooh and say look Tigger is jumping, but Tigger says he is **bouncing**. "Parag what do we bounce," so we get to introduce the next target action word! Now the target word shifts us to a new activity basketball! We taught Parag all the colors by bouncing various colored balloons.

When I learned to speak Spanish, I was able to communicate because I had a good repertoire of vocabulary. Gradually, I was able to use them in sentences. If I am thirsty and can say "sed", Spanish speaking people understand that I am thirsty. So vocabulary is the first step to communication and a gateway to language acquisition. Keeping this in mind we designed various ways to teach vocabulary to Parag. First was recognition of objects. We made him look at three dimensional objects, never more than five at a time, during the teaching process. First we asked him to touch it, or to give it. This is **receptive** checking and then we showed him one object at a time, and asked him "what is this," this is **expressive** checking. The same goes for picture flash cards. We also review some of these informally outside the classroom. When we go for a walk, I may ask him to show me: rock, gate, grass, brick, swing, bug etc. Informal teaching has to be fun, the primary purpose is a pleasant walk, teaching has to be so subtle that Parag should not figure out that he is still being taught.

After the objects and the flash cards are mastered, Parag has to categorize, like match the pants with clothes, apple with fruits, hammer with tools. We check and if the concept is mastered by putting clothes, fruits and tools together, he has to take the object out and put them in separate baskets, each basket has the category written on it: clothes, tools and fruits. We used to do matching, through flash cards also, we said "put with the same," and he matched the similar things. The practical application of this task is that he puts away the dishes from the dish washer by matching them and then stacks them in an appropriate place in the cabinets. It is mind boggling to see his precision in matching the cutlery! What more can a parent ask, a communication skill also metamorphosing into a life skill.

After doing the flash cards, we also made our own worksheet to reiterate and extend the concepts. Parag has twenty spelling words per week. He reviews them every day for two weeks and on a Thursday, he takes a test. Five words out of twenty are maintenance words, he has done them before, and we are checking to see if he can still retrieve them. Parag is allowed to look at the board on which the words are written. After all, he needs to help himself when he is stuck. Initially we directed him to look at the spelling word that he was stuck on, and he copied it. Now he does that on his own. On the day of the test we erase all the words from the board. After he takes the test, the words, that he gets wrong go on the board again. Once he masters these words, it goes on a big pocket chart and becomes a part of a word wall. This way these learned words are visually always there and every morning during calendar time (asking day, date, month and what kind of weather it is), the therapist reviews some of those words as well.

Parag has no problem in communicating his wants and needs in the present tense but has hard time with past and future tense. So to teach it in a concrete way. Every Tuesday, he has to write what he is going to do on Wednesday, his day out from school, essentially his grocery day. So the teacher guides him to write: what they will do **tomorrow**. Then on Thursday he has to write what they did **yesterday** and read it. This enables him to have a short conversation, which is prompted by the teacher. This way we know that he is getting the scheduled repetition of the skill taught. We do other things to enhance his recall in the past tense or future tense. After reading a story about "a little duckling"; we may go to feed bread crumbs to the ducks by the river. We do the same. We talk about what we are going to do, and after feeding the ducks, we talk about what we did. This is a spur of the moment decision made by the teacher to further enhance the concepts and bring an element of fun by having a short outing. Regularity and repetition are the key to teaching Parag.

Recently, I gave Parag a spelling test and I was pretty amused to see that he had invented a new way to write cucumber. He had written "qcumber." Talk about sounding out letters in a word! If given the chance, I wouldn't mind writing the same spelling, because it makes more sense. If American English is all about simplifying British English: Ok for okay, check for cheque, why not qcumber for cucumber? Imagine how difficult it must be for children with autism to understand why "put" and "but" sound different!

We also teach vocabulary by labeling the surroundings with sticky notes. For example, when we are targeting to teach him all the things in the restroom. We label the sink, faucet, commode, shower, mirror basically all the things in there. We take him in the bathroom and ask him to "point to or touch" a particular object in the bathroom. Once he does that, then we ask him to say what it is. To see if he has mastered those we gradually take away the sticky note and if he tells us the correct response, then that object is considered mastered and we go on asking it with other stuff but without the visual cue of the sticky note. This way he gets to learn both receptively and expressively. This contextual teaching is extended in the classroom through the picture flashcard. We gather picture flashcards pertaining to the bathroom and the objects there. We also put soap, soap case, loofah, shampoo, comb, towel etc. small things in the basket. This way he is exposed to real three dimensional objects. Then there are computer programs which do the discreet trial training for the same. This computer program teaches the same concept but breaks it down where a child is successful with repeated practice. Positive feedbacks are used as reinforcers, which are delivered when the child selects the right answer. When he/she does not get the answer in a couple of trials then the computer automatically reduces the complexity. These kinds of computer programs are very effective for drill and practice. In teaching Parag we have tried to incorporate a variety of ways to teach the same concepts. This makes the teaching and learning process not boring. Otherwise anything that is based on drill and practice becomes boring very fast. It is important to teach in a variety of ways and through different media. Once learning is not boring then the resistance to learn and behavioral problems also go down.

We teach Parag to pronounce and enunciate loudly and clearly. That is one of the primary teaching goals. This is important because we who are involved with Parag understand what he is saying even when what he says may not be clear. It can be difficult for others to understand him. For example he sometimes says "showee" for shower when he is asking for permission to take shower. I understand but at the same time correct him. Seldom I don't understand what Parag is saying and that is the time I ask him to "show me." Once he shows me, I am able to figure out what he is saying and then I make time to teach him to say it properly with the right pronunciation and enunciation. This process of incidental learning helps in teaching things contextually.

I have told you Parag is smart and cheeky. Parag likes to mix a spoon full of sugar in the milk and drink it. Lot of times he says "spoon. " Well, he is not asking for a spoon, he is actually asking me for a "spoon full of sugar". When I say tell me what you really want, then he says "sugar." Parag purposely avoids saying "sugar" because he knows he will not get it from me. Sometimes to make him talk, I say "ok if you say the whole sentence I will give you sugar." Then he is instantly motivated and he says the sentence "I want to eat spoon full of sugar." I am stating this because incidental teaching and contextual teaching are powerful tools to teach communications. This is an example that shows that things that we teach formally get expanded and Parag uses communication skills for his own benefit.

I have also noticed that when doing a flash card with Parag if the question is not specific then Parag gives a nonspecific answer. It may be the right answer but that is not what I am looking for, because I am aiming for a more specific answer. Recently, I was checking his recognition of objects both through flash cards and three dimensional objects. I showed him a flash card and asked him "what is this?" Parag promptly replied food; the answer was right but not what I was looking for. So I said "yes, what food?" Then he said "rice" and that was the answer I wanted. When I showed him the flashcard with duck, he said bird and when I asked what kind of bird, he said "duck." I remember one time the behaviorist who used to come to check Parag's progress was showing the flash cards to Parag. She showed him the picture of a glass filled with juice. She asked him what it was. Parag promptly replied glass. She said "no" and moved to another card. I intervened and asked her if I could show him the card. She did and I showed Parag the flashcard but changed the question "what is in the glass?" He promptly replied "juice." The reason I am relating this incident is because if we want specific answers the questions have to be specific. Also, it must have been confusing for Parag to understand why the behaviorist said "no" when he was giving her the right answer. I figured out that she wanted Parag to say juice and when Parag did not answer thus, she moved on to the next flashcard. We sometimes are so set in our ways of teaching that we do not pause and analyze our flaws of our teaching methods. The only reason I was able to detect this was because I knew the thought process behind Parag's answer. We all know same question can have multiple right answers. Everyone has various perspectives in seeing the same thing. So the question has to be right before expecting the right answer!

Recently after giving Parag a cookie I asked "what do you say?" I was expecting "thank you" for an answer instead Parag said, "Give me." I said, "try again." He thought and then said "Give me please." I could not help smiling because "please" is something we remind him to say. After that I asked him to say "thank you" which he did. Parag's answer was right, it was different from what I was expecting. Also I don't like to say "no" or "wrong" when Parag tries and does not give the expected answer. **We should always encourage children for trying. It is positive when we say "good trying, try again or yes, think of another answer." Every attempt and trial should be praised/reinforced.**

Parag remembers the skills that we teach him. He also applies them appropriately in the right context. The big blessing is that Parag generalizes his skills in various settings. I believe a gradual increase in communication skills has made Parag socially more adept. He is able to reach out to people and convey his wants and needs and they are able to understand. This makes him happy. **Communication leads to social inclusion and acceptance for kids with autism**. The goal of all these skills and activities is to enhance communication skills, comprehension and awareness of the surroundings. Variety in teaching strategies also helps in assimilation and generalization.

Exercise and personal grooming

Personal grooming and hygiene along with exercise are intertwined with good health for everyone. Grooming is essential for all children, more so for special needs children. Research based study shows that epilepsy and infectious diseases are the most common causes of death for individuals with autism spectrum disorder. Accidental deaths in the younger population are often due to drowning and suffocation. This information gives awareness to the caregivers and also prepares them for preventive measures and reduces associated risks of death. It is obvious that to avoid infections, being clean personally and keeping the surroundings neat and clean reduces the risk of infections for everyone; it is the best course of prevention for the children with autism spectrum disorder.

To have good health and hygiene is an asset that increases the quality of life. Parag takes Risperdal, to help him calm down. The side effect is weight gain. I got concerned when Parag's became overweight and I was not sure how to tackle this. This medicine makes him hungry. Parag's schedule is such that he gets to play outside, ride a bike and swim but these activities were not enough. Particularly in winter he gains weight, because all the outside activities come to a standstill.

I started getting worried once he hit the 250 pounds. He is six feet tall but still he looked overweight. Research shows that obesity can lead to lot of ailments such as high blood pressure and diabetes, heart attack, stroke and even cancer. I want Parag to be healthy and since he does not know how to take care of his health, it is my job to guide him and put him on a healthy diet. After all, he eats what I cook.

I started making him walk on the treadmill at the pace of brisk walk for an hour and a half in the beginning and then tapered it down to an hour. This was not easy, because about two years ago, he had fallen from it, and he would look at the treadmill and say ohoo (hurt). I patiently tried to make him see me do the treadmill first and would tell him it is fun. In the beginning I did not ask him to get on the treadmill. Once, he started standing, beside me while I was still on the machine. I knew he would give it a try and so he did. I said Parag "mom is done, you go and he got on it!

When Parag walks on the treadmill, we put the TV on. This makes his exercise less boring. After all who likes to walk on the treadmill? We also take Parag for a long walk by the lake, which is approximately a three mile trail. It is a very pretty sight to see Parag running like a colt, who has just figured out how to run!

I have also reduced his food portion size. I give him teaspoon to eat his dinner, that way it takes longer for him to finish his food and his satiety center gets satisfied. I also make him drink at least two to three glasses of water while he is eating. If he gets hungry between the meals, we give him fruits. He has lost sixty pounds in the last eight months. This strategy is working for him. Parag has run couple of five kilometer runs. The first race he came second in his age group! I am so proud of him and we run 5k's together as a family. We have joined the local runners club. I hope all of us can run a half marathon together, that will be a family achievement! Running is easier for Parag because it does not have cumbersome rules like other sports, all he has to do is take off and reach the finish line!

Parag's health is important and so is the health of the entire family. Caregivers have to take care of themselves, so they are able to take care of others. It is the same thing they say on the airplane, in time of emergency, put the oxygen mask on yourself first and then on the kid. To provide help, you should be in good condition to do so. The same concept applies, when you have to take care of a kid with autism. The entire family needs to be healthy both physically and mentally. I realized early on that in taking care of Parag I had to be as fit as possible. I started exercising regularly. Like gardening it gave me physical strength and mental solace. If for some unforeseen reasons I get off the routine, it haunts me until I straighten up my act.

Pranav, my husband, also reacted to Parag's autism in his unique and protective way. He became worried about finances, because raising a child with autism is a big financial commitment. I saw that man transform from a happy go lucky person to a workaholic. In this process, he ignored his health and gained weight. However, he too realized that he has to take care of himself before he can take care of anyone else. He follows an exercise regimen and loves running marathons. He has inspired me to run marathons too. We have started hiking together and it is an amazing experience to connect with Nature. I sometimes wonder would we have done all this if Parag did not have autism.

Ankur, my elder son joined the cross-fit gym which help him build his physical and mental toughness. He used to find comfort in food to deal with his stress. This time he exercised and followed a diet and has lost 58 pounds. Now he watches what he eats and tries to eat healthy. He is trying to be responsible and have discipline.

I feel that exercising has made all of us more upbeat. We all are able to handle our challenges better. We also connect by talking about what exercise we did and how we are going to meet our goals. Best of all we laugh together. Pranav, being a physician, is especially concerned with Parag's hygiene habits. He often reiterates that it is of utmost importance to teach Parag to take care of his body and oral health. All this information made me teach Parag to groom himself. It is like reflex now, that after waking up, Parag uses the restroom and shower. He then dresses up and brushes his teeth, combs his hair, puts his sandals on and is ready for the school to begin. It has been a lot of work for us and the caregivers/teachers to teach him all this to a point where it has become a habit or in other words he is conditioned.

The teaching process is pretty intricate because there are so many mini steps to it that it is hard to write and describe; one finds a solution while working on it. To teach Parag to dress on his own, I had to show him the tag on the shirt and say, "tag goes in the back and inside," with repetition he became aware of looking at the tag and then turning around the shirt so that tag was in the back. Buttoning his shirt was something we made him learn. It too was a process of making him look and see what he was doing. He wears briefs (underwear), with the pouch in the front which I call a pocket, so I made him look and told him "pocket goes in the front." By showing, he understood what I meant by the words "back" and "front." We showed him how to zip his pants and jackets. We had to make him look at locking the zip of the jacket together before he could pull it all the way up. For the socks, we got the ones which has different color on the heel, so he knew; the colored portion should fit on the heel. I also bought tube socks where he could wear the socks any way he pleases. The shoes he wears don't have laces because we are still teaching him to tie the shoe lace. The reason he has not mastered it is because I did not think it was very important at the early stages of homeschooling. There were many things we were teaching Parag along with tackling his behaviors. I felt it was not one of the most important things that we were dealing with at that time. Parag could wear shoes without shoe laces and it was fine. Making Parag wear tube socks is the same mentality. The thought process is to simplify. Tackle it when other important skills, skills essential for survival are mastered. We are teaching him to tie the shoe laces now because we have more time for refining on his grooming skills. We are out of that phase of tantrums and behavior problems and that allows us to allocate our time to more refined grooming skills. The initial teachings were essential grooming skills.

We made him brush his teeth. He had to put the tooth paste on the brush, spread it otherwise he used to eat it, then we had to show him hand over hand what to do. He has to rinse once the timer went off and then use nonalcoholic mouth wash. He also has to put away everything properly; to keep the work area neat is also a part of grooming. In the shower he had to use a loofah and body bath to scrub himself and we showed him how. The same went for shampoo. Once he came out of the shower, he had to dry himself off and we showed him how. All this took about two years of consistent and persistent training every single day to instill these grooming and hygiene skills as habits. Using the restroom and wiping himself well was a hand over hand thing, which I had done during the toilet training process, then letting him wipe on his own. Eventually, he could do this on his own. Washing hands with the soap after using the restroom and drying his hands was a teaching process as well.

Parag loves to have a haircut now but it was a nightmare in the beginning. Parag would be crying and writhing. He was scared of the electric clippers. We asked the barber, to use scissors and then use the clippers at the end to trim. All the while we were trying to talk to Parag and trying to calm him down. Gradually, Parag was not scared of the hair cut or the clippers.

We are teaching Parag to shave and he loves the attention. We make him look in the mirror and then hand over hand guide him to shave. We are easing on the prompt because he is taking the razor from us and wanting to shave on his own. We respect his independent spirit and watch him while he is shaving, we draw his attention to the spot he misses. We still cut Parag's nails because he won't cut on his own. He is scared to cut his nails. There was a point in time when he did not want to part with his overgrown nails and once I cut them, he would cry and ask me to put it back again. I am so glad those days are over! I have not come around to figuring this out as how to take away the phobia. The reason is I have to deal with cutting the nails only once in two weeks, most of the time Ankur or Pranav cut Parag's nails. I believe teaching cutting nails will go in the list of things to be taught, once some skills that are presently in the list get mastered. Once the skill goes on the report card, our individualized education plan, then the skills get special and regular attention. We chalk out what we are going to do, how and when we will teach the task. These are daily living skills and life skills, so they will be taught contextually.

There is an overwhelming amount of teaching going on with Parag, in all his deficit areas. We have to prioritize which skills and tasks we are going to teach first. Dealing with too many tasks at one time does not give the desired results and also leads to dissipation of energy. When we bite off more than we can chew, we choke. This is exactly what happens when we start working on too many goals at one time. When we don't see results, both the teacher and the student feel disappointment and setback. I have made this mistake and I believe **it is better to be slow and steady with lots of practice and drills.** Once we take over the teaching of a skill then repetition and regular practice becomes the norm. Teaching basic grooming skills was tedious and challenging but has paid off. It has released us from assisting him. It also gives me the satisfaction that the habits of grooming and hygiene will make Parag healthier and less prone to infections. One of the good things with Parag is he likes to be clean, he does not like to sweat, so after playing outside or exercising, he takes shower on his own and changes his clothes.

Keeping the surroundings clean is also part of hygiene. I have taught Parag to put things back where they belong. He had to place all his toys back where they went. I have taught him everything has an allotted space and it should go there. Parag has this obsessive compulsive disorder to be clean and neat, which helps with the grooming and hygiene process. He will make sure that he puts his washed clothes in his closet and the dirty clothes in the hamper. These were things I taught him without even thinking that I was training him to become neat. I am happy with the results. I have described his obsessive compulsive disorder, in the chapter: Parag's obsessive compulsive disorder. That chapter goes in depth about how Parag keeps his environment and surrounding neat and also some training processes. However, his innate nature to be clean and orderly makes it easy to keep my house organized and clean!

We have also taught Parag that we dress differently with the change of seasons. I change his wardrobe according to the seasonal changes. Parag instinctively perceives the need of different types of clothes with the temperature change. In the winter he starts wearing jackets and sweaters because he is cold. Many times he stands on the air conditioning vent to be toasty and cozy from the warm air coming out of it. During summer he feels hot, he takes two to three showers per day or prefers to be in the swimming pool to cool off.

It is important to teach special needs children basic personal grooming as early as possible. We can then go on refining and adding to those skills. I do believe it is better to keep it simple in the beginning. There are tons of clothes and gadgets available to assist special needs people. Special types of clothes are lot easier to wear and take off, it may have Velcro instead of buttons. It may not have tags so it does not have a back and a front. These are advertised as "adaptive clothing." These special clothes, shoes and specialized gadgets are life savers for children who are challenged in fine motor skills or have a lot of difficulty with hand eye coordination.

There are many videos and DVDS' in the market that visually teach personal grooming. There are tons of programs on Public Broadcasting Systems (PBS) on personal grooming for children. These also help the children with autism and other children to learn from watching. These programs show how the wardrobe changes with the change of seasons and why we need to wear woolens in the winter and lighter clothes in the summer. Essential oral hygiene and taking showers and baths are very tastefully modeled by the children and in a fun way too.

I chose to teach Parag to wear regular clothes and shoes because I knew he could learn to do so. It is easier to shop for Parag's clothes because he wears what the general population wears. This also gives us the opportunity to go to the stores together and shop, an experience both of us enjoy. Parag goes shopping for his clothes with his teacher also because she follows the trendy stuff and fashion. We do want him to be upbeat and fashionable. The children with autism need to be neat and clean and well-dressed not just to avoid infections but this also makes them socially more acceptable. This mantra works for everyone. Being well groomed increases their social acceptance and social adaptability.

Vacation, Recreation and Respite

Research shows that all parents endure stress but studies also show that parents of children with developmental disabilities, like autism, experience depression and anxiety even more. The challenges to juggle their life between crucial support services, financial strain of therapies and relentless worries as well as uncertainty of the future takes a huge toll on the parents. It is not surprising that they start showing signs of depression.

Recreation is an important opportunity for the family to rejuvenate and spend quality time with each other. It is a much needed fuel for the mind and body in general and absolutely a must for a family with a child with autism. Taking a break from the demanding tempo of life is a recharging and revitalizing experience. To do this doesn't mean taking a long vacation; actually a small trip is as enjoyable. Going to the restaurant, movies and games are all part of this. The point is to relax and feel "I am ready to handle anything that comes my way." In the beginning, I tried to involve Parag in every leisure activity. My zeal to make Parag socially adept took over, since the decision was emotional, it had an innate flaw. I soon realized this was not healthy. Balance is the key. Every family member needs to have special time with each other.

We take Parag to the movies, football games and to restaurants. He loves going to birthday parties. He likes blowing balloons and we have made him the designated balloon blower at these parties. An exercise for his lungs! This is a pleasant break from the routine for all of us. However, there are times we send Parag with the teacher to a movie. My husband and I go out with Ankur. Sometimes my husband and I go out or spend time with friends. These breaks, I believe are even more important than going out on a trip or vacation. The reason is these are small but much needed respites from the mundane routine. Sometimes when we take a long break, it becomes harder for us to pick up from where we had left off. The pace of the home school gets broken. The small breaks and outings are like nourishment for the mind. Afterward I am ready to handle the next day with energy and enthusiasm.

We took Parag to Italy in 2007, it was a bus tour. The first day, all the tourists traveling in the bus met in a conference room to introduce each other. My husband introduced Parag and let everyone know he is autistic. This is one of the most memorable tours; for once people knew about Parag, they just spoiled him rotten. Of course, Parag loved all the attention he got. Parag thrives on that. It is funny that he remembers the Italian gesture of being upset. Italians flick their finger under the chin to show they are annoyed. It means "get lost", and is used in Belgium, France, North Italy and Tunisia. Parag was listening to the tour guide who showed the gesture and since then he has picked that gesture and uses it, to show he is not happy.

I had read that autistic children do not imitate till you teach them. This is a misconception that autistic people do not learn from their environment on their own. The above incident is an example of learning through observation. Environment and exposure gives everyone, including children with autism the opportunity to learn by sheer osmosis. It is a passive process, one does not realize but it rubs off on them. I agree that one can increase the pace of a learning process through imitation of behaviors and gestures by modeling and active teaching.

We had a great family trip to Savannah, Georgia, a beautiful colonial town. I remember one incident worth sharing. We got on a trolley, which gives a tour to eighty different places where scenes for the movies were filmed in Savannah. I am such a fan of the movie Forest Gump that I was eager to see the bench where Tom Hanks has said the memorable lines "Life is like a box of chocolates, you never know what you are going to get." We all were waiting for the tour to start but our bus driver and the tour guide was welcoming but garrulous. She was so animated that, she went on and on for at least for forty minutes to an hour. All of a sudden, Parag got up and said to her "no more, all done, go outside." We tried to persuade Parag to sit down but Parag refused, he was determined to avoid listening to our tour guide, we apologized and got off the trolley. We marched back to the hotel, my husband said Parag just saved us from the relentless rambling of the tour guide; we all laughed and agreed unanimously. We had to walk our way to the hotel and that is one of the most memorable walks, for we got to see all the beautiful homes and parks and the first Girl Scout National center. So, what I am trying to say is sometimes things don't work out the way we have planned things, but if we are flexible, and find fun, then you get to experience it anyway. I also feel, that missing that trolley for the movie tour, has given us an incentive to visit this place again and to build more memories. The experience has also made us wiser; we will board the trolley, when the briefing is over!

One time we all went to Disney World in Florida. We were having a blast exploring the Magic Kingdom and Animal kingdom. Parag got hungry and asked for food. All the food stalls were jam packed with people waiting in the ques. We were crossing a picnic area and pacifying Parag that we will get him something to eat. Well, Parag had lost patience with us, so he decided to join a group of people who were picnicking, he found the corner spot of their bench empty, so Parag took off his hand from mine, and very proudly perched himself at the empty spot and then tells the family "coke". They were amused and when we apologized, they were gracious enough to include all of us. We excused ourselves, but Parag by that time had got a coke, said bye to them and walked away very contented. This was a learning experience for us, as caregivers. After this incident, I keep snacks and something to drink always available.

I remember an incident at Biltmore estate. Parag was around five then. We were having a tour of the place. In one room there is a grand piano. Before we knew Parag ducked under the rope barrier and sat on the stool and started playing songs. We were flustered, before security guys could intervene, we dragged our Mozart away. Now, I remember this incident with a smile but when it was happening, believe me I was almost about to have a massive heart attack. After this incident, we became strict to where he can play piano. We allowed him to play at friend's house but not in the club, a public place. He had to learn and we learned too. As I have stated before a lot of times an incident triggers an intervention plan.

Recently, we went to Punta- Cana. Parag was sitting by the window; he was fascinated to see the plane take off. He pulled down the blinds and after a while put it up to peek and check at the status, if we were still flying. Parag would pull the blind again and look at us laughing and starry eyed. Even though he has flown many times, it was this time he really connected with the experience. The expression on his face was a mixture of bewilderment, fascination and sheer joy. When he was a toddler, he was more interested in getting coke and candies from the air hostess. The moment he saw an air hostess, he would ask for a coke. This vacation was one of the most relaxing vacations. Parag was so happy for all his favorite food was available all the time. He gobbled ice cream, chicken fingers and French fries, no wonder he gained six pounds in four days. We have taken him on car trips to Grand Canyon and the

Grand Tetons. After a helicopter ride over the Grand canyon, Parag was fascinated by the helicopter. He lead us to the souvenir shop there and asked for the biggest helicopter for his memento collection.

He loves to visit his grandparents at Auburn, Alabama. I always warn him in the car to behave but Parag is honest he tells me outright "no, naughty boy." That is, "I will be a naughty boy at the grand parents." I find his honesty so charming and disarming at the same time. The reason he says this is, he is ready to invade grandma's pantry and overjoyed to get his way with them. He is able to show us how powerful he is when he has loving allies, his grandparents. Parag lies down on the sofa and munches chips and eats ice cream away! Grandparents are a big respite for us too, because visiting them is a break from our routine.

There are vacations we plan with Ankur. There are two reasons for this; first, we want to spend time with Ankur our older son, exclusively. Our big chunk of time is taken by Parag and in running his school smoothly. So it is important for us to enjoy Ankur's company and special vacations with him. Secondly, these vacations like checking out the ruins of Machu-Pichu in Peru or the hiking trip to Pikes peaks in Colorado are too demanding and precarious for Parag. When we plan a vacation like these, we make arrangements for Parag to stay at home. Parag's teacher, looks after him. She is like another mother to him. She and her family love Parag. We know that he is well taken care of in our absence and this is a big relief and blessing for all of us.

While planning a vacation with Parag, we make sure to pack some of his favorite things, like his i-Pad, so he can listen to his favorite songs and watch his movies, if he desires. Parag's medicines are an absolute must. After the Disney world incident, where he deserted us for food, I always pack some of his favorite snacks. The good thing that has happened with taking all these vacation and trips is that Parag, unlike many autistic children, is not bothered by change in the routine. He actually looks forward to a break from his routine. We lovingly call him Marco Polo, the explorer.

To me an hour for myself in the gym or some time to read a book is very satisfying. It has taken me time to inculcate the thought process that Parag is in good hands and the person with whom I have left him with is extremely capable and trustworthy. It is important for the parents and caregivers to feel that their special needs kid will be well taken care of even when they are not around. Mental respite is as important as physical respite. In raising a kid with autism, the nuance of balance becomes crystal clear. I believe that small breaks from routines are as recharging as a long vacation, actually sometimes it works better than a long vacation. The reason is long vacation breaks the tempo of skill teaching to the kids with autism. Going to the movies, games or just hanging out with friends and families is a great way to recuperate and less expensive than a vacation. Vacation requires planning both the time availability and financial feasibility. If parents and caregivers can come up with an inbuilt system of respites and recreation for themselves, in their daily routine, that will be tremendously energy boosting and keep them going like the energizer bunny!

What happens when school is not running?

If the teacher must be away, then how is Parag's day? Well, the answer is how is my schedule? The ultimate backup teacher is the mom. Ideally, I like to spend at least three hours in the classroom with him and teach him. Generally I spend time with Parag on Fridays and this gives me an opportunity to teach him whatever we are working on like comprehension through reading and vocabulary training (the teaching of these has been described in the chapter "Teaching communication"). I also address anything that the teacher has asked me to teach additionally.

Most of the time after getting ready, Parag goes to the classroom on his own; he is conditioned that way since he was about six years old. He realizes, since the teacher is not there, he is at leisure to do what he likes. It is his fun day. Most of the time, he may play Wii, listen to music and dance along with the songs, or watch his favorite movies. I can see him from the downstairs TV, for his classroom is monitored by a camera. Parag is able to engage himself meaningfully! I can do my chores and still keep an eye on him. It also is a good monitoring device; it helps to keep an eye on the classroom activities. If I have errands, he accompanies me and loves to play hooky from the school. For example, if I have to go to the bank he comes with me. This outing gives him an opportunity to show off his social skills. I ask him to sit down, while I do my stuff. He loves flipping through the pages of a magazine. The same way, he could be taken along to the grocery store. At home if I have to cook, then he sometimes does puzzles or listens to music. Sometimes he will just sit around and watches me cook.

The only thing I cannot do on a day like this is go to my dental or doctor's appointment. I don't like to take Parag to a doctor's clinic, not because he won't be well behaved but I don't want him to be exposed to germs and sick people. To keep him in good health and hygiene is always mandatory. When Parag is sick he acts like a baby. He demands my undivided attention and lots of tender loving care(TLC).

During a holiday, like the Fourth of July, Halloween, Thanks giving and Christmas, Parag is off from the school. He spends time with the family, doing what everyone is doing. For example, we barbecue on the fourth of July (American Independence Day), we just pig out, swim, play games, watch movies and in the evening watch the fireworks show organized by the City of Gadsden. On Thanksgiving, we watch football games and of course have a grand meal in the evening. When Parag and Ankur were young, they went to trick or treat on Halloween but once these boys turned into teen agers, they stopped doing that, instead they wait in the house for the "trick or treaters" and give them candies. Parag loves it either way, the fact being, he is able to eat candies! It is the same way on Christmas Eve, we have sumptuous meal and on Christmas morning, Parag gets to open up his gifts, like all of us. The point is if the school is not running on a holiday, then Parag is doing what all other family members are doing.

Breaking from the routine is vital for Parag. I read that many children with autism are not able to handle change in routine. His daily schedule changes too, so that there is no regimental routine. Parag's adjusting to the change of routine has proven to be a boon. He is not only accepting but he likes it too. I am so thankful for his flexibility and adaptability. So if there is a break in the regular routine, it is not only manageable but enjoyable for both Parag and me. It has taken me time to reach this point and make it work. **The first thing I had to learn was to accept that the day will be different than what I had planned previously.** Second, was if I deal with the day with a positive frame of mind, it will be a very satisfying day for both Parag and me. In the evening, at dinner time we share how every ones day went. Parag and I have something different to share. At the same time I want the readers to know this is not a norm. I cannot have Parag off schedule for long, then it won't be fun. This is a once in a while thing which breaks the monotony!

Parag's Obsessive Compulsive Disorders

Children with Autism display many kinds of obsessive compulsive disorders. They display repetitive behaviors and vocalizations. Generally people who have an obsessive compulsive disorder, are aware of their obsessive compulsive behaviors and want to control it, so they seek help. People with Autism Spectrum disorder, are not bothered by these behaviors. On the contrary they seem to be comforted or soothed by them. When Parag was a toddler, he loved to line up small cars and stare at them. He also loved to twirl stuff and look at them in excitement, he hyperextended his body when he stared at the rotating object. Once I took away these cars or the twirling toys, he would get upset and throw a big tantrum. The more he played like that, he did not want to interact with anyone and he became more resistant to give those toys up. I figured out that Parag likes to play in this ritualistic manner and I knew, if these OCD behaviors were not addressed it would lead to strong resistance from Parag and eventually, manifest as aggressive behavior.

I intervened with determination. The best solution I came to tackle this with was to use these toys as reinforcers. They were used during the early phase of the home school. This is how the fading was done. If Parag wanted the toys, he could have them for a while, once he performed a task for me or the teacher, while we were teaching. There were times in between these sessions that Parag threw tantrums to get his toys. Well, all I did was to stay calm. Looking back I don't know from where I got that ability to withhold. Once he realized that the only way to get those was to do what was asked of him, his tantrums reduced in frequency and eventually faded. The pairing of these reinforcers with praises, compliments and other reinforcers like television time, listening to his favorite music or time to play on the computer eventually eliminated these obsessive compulsive behaviors. These behaviors were interfering in his normal day to day life activities and interactions. It took almost two years to fade them away completely.

Any object that will trigger his obsessive compulsive behaviors is not used in the school anymore. We don't want him to regress. The regression is not instant but exposing him to these objects could make him want them again and with greater fervor. The objects that triggers the obsessive compulsive behavior in kids with autism is analogous to drugs for drug addicts or alcohol for alcoholics relapsing. To keep them clean from the addictive habit we should not expose them recurrently to an environment that triggers the behavior.

The fact that we tackled and got rid of his debilitating obsessive compulsive disorder behaviors early on was a very smart move. I know a kid with autism, who loves to play the same video games for hours. When asked to stop, it leads to aggressive behaviors. As these children grow, they become stronger and then to stop these obsessive compulsive behaviors, require an effort beyond imagination. As I have said before, it is like an addiction for the children with Autism disorder. The more we let perseverating (repetition of insistent and redundant behavior) and unsocial ritualistic behavior happen the more they will want to engage in such behaviors, until it manifests itself as a nightmare of aggressive behavior problems. Some medicines may help to calm them down but the behavioral interventions have to go hand in hand. **The earlier the intervention is initiated and implemented the better.**

I hope that some parents who are still struggling with obsessive ritualistic behaviors of their kid with autism may be able to apply what we did with Parag. They can use the objects and toys that their child is obsessively attached to as primary reinforcers just as we did with Parag. Then gradually fade them away. During the training, fading happens both by reducing the time that they can have their self-stimulatory toys and also by replacing those with other appropriate activities and objects.

Parag sometimes gets obsessed with one shirt or pair of pants and wants to wear the same ones all the time. Right now it is a tee-shirt that his cousin has given him, which says Harvard Business School. I don't think he is wearing this tee-shirt for the prestigious label, but he is wearing it because red is his favorite color. Then again, I could be wrong for you never know what Parag is thinking! It could be totally about the emblem. There was a phase when he loved to gaze at emblems like CNN, APT etc. displayed at the corner of the television, while the television program was going on or in the magazines. He was also fascinated by the numbers on the credit cards. So it could be either the color or the emblem in the tee-shirt or both! When this phenomenon occurs, all I do is hide those for a while. He looks for them in every closet and also asks for them. My answer is simple, "if you can find it, you can wear it". When he does not find them, after looking for them in every single closet in the house, he wears what is available in his closet. After a month or so I put it back in his closet. By then, the obsession seems to have subsided. This has also occurred with certain kinds of University of Alabama pajamas, the same happened to the pajamas. I played Houdini with them as well.

The interesting thing is that some of Parag's obsessive compulsive disorder behaviors have been channeled to work for him and us. He is neat and organized and likes to keep things a certain way. When he was young I would make him keep all his toys in a basket after he had played with them. He had to keep all his stuff where it belonged. Now if he sees anything not in its proper place, Parag makes sure that he puts it away. For example, he will keep all the pencils and pens in the holder. Parag puts the remotes neatly on one side of the coffee table. The places where I have the holder for the remotes, he puts them there. Parag likes to close all the cabinet doors and I like it, for I definitely like my cabinet doors closed. Parag does not like pillows on the sofa to be out of place, so if they are he will fix it. If you find my house very orderly and organized, Parag is chipping in big time in it too. Actually, these obsessive compulsive behaviors have proved to be helpful both for Parag and us. It is great to have a son who likes to help keep the house spic and span.

The gist is that not all obsessive compulsive behaviors are detrimental and debilitating toward appropriate social development. The ones that lead to ritualistic behavior, start interfering with the day to day functioning and hinder appropriate social interactions have to be eradicated early on. In case of Parag his being neat and orderly works for him and us!

School rules and decorum

Punctuality is essential. Everyone involved with school has to be at work on time and cannot be absent from work until and unless it is a real emergency. The fact that the school is run at home does not mean a teacher can be lax about her own attendance in teaching Parag. The time card is there so everyone working with Parag has to clock in and clock out, this way their hours of work automatically gets recorded. Also, there is backup system. If the teacher is not able to come, then I am the backup. I like to be told beforehand that way I am mentally prepared to teach. I have to be mentally ready to take over and this gives me time to deal with other household stuff that needs to be taken care off. I organize everything, in such a way that I am not only physically free but mentally free as well. The fruitful interactions and teaching happens, when I am totally present in what I am doing.

Phone calls cannot be entertained in the classroom. If it is very important, the teacher has to go out of the classroom to do so. Parag's lessons are very interactive and disruptions like phone calls take away the tempo. Moreover, any classroom runs effectively, when time is managed optimally, by following the schedule. Time management is next to impossible. When we entertain phone calls while teaching. In the beginning many of my friends did not understand, why it was so hard for me to entertain their phone calls, while I am teaching. I believe they feel, it is a home school, I have leeway to teach when I want. I don't and neither does anyone teaching Parag. I don't know if they understand but by now they have accepted it.

The school has certain decorum. A dress code is one of them. Every one dresses comfortably. No one can be in the formal classroom in pajamas, that is in the morning sessions between 9:00 to 2:30. I feel when I am in pajamas, my brain goes into the resting mode and I am not alert and agile. School requires alertness of mind and body. During the early phases of the program, I realized that when the teachers see me in pajamas they too get lax, after all the school is run at home. There is a dress code for every environment, and Parag needs to learn that as well. It would be ludicrous to see someone in a formal suit at the beach!

Many times, children with special needs who are home schooled are in pajamas or their certain favorite clothes all the time at home. They become so conditioned to wearing those that they want to go out in them. Trying to make them wear an appropriate outfit becomes hard and sometimes leads to physical resistance. I know someone, who has autism and resists wearing other clothes, except pajamas. The parents are so scared of his resistance that they take him to church in pajamas. This made me decide that Parag will always be appropriately dressed for different occasions. He can wear Pajamas for his informal school that is when his buddies come to play with him in the afternoon around three thirty. However, he changes into his exercise clothes before he walks on the treadmill. If Parag is going to swim in the pool, he has to change into swimming trunks. Parag does not resist changing into different outfits because this was instilled in him at an early age. Parag goes outside, to restaurants and games properly dressed for the occasion. This makes him blend in with the crowd and not draw unnecessary attention. I feel that when children with special needs are dressed appropriately and are groomed properly, people accept them with greater ease.

The rule of being properly dressed is mandatory for teachers also. As a teacher, in this kind of a classroom, I should be able to sit on the floor or run outside and play. I remember an incident when Parag was about six.One of the teachers was working in the classroom with Parag, and when I came in to see, how everything was going, I noticed that the teacher's panties were showing through her mini skirt. I asked her to sit properly for I did not want Parag to see that. What amazed me was her reply; she said that Parag did not understand. That was the only teacher in eighteen years that I had to let go. A person who believes that her student does not understand cannot and should not teach. **The dress code is important but the mindset is even more important.**

The other thing, I always ask the teacher to do is not come to teach in a bad mood or bring emotional problems to work. The teacher has to be mentally present in the classroom, otherwise their mood resonates and it leads to unnecessary behavioral problems by the student. If the teacher is distracted, it is not fair to the student. This is true for any teacher, more so a special education teacher. I feel all teachers have to learn to compartmentalize their lives but the need for this is even greater for the teachers who have to teach special needs students. **Once inside the classroom, it is the teacher's job to turn a bad day into a good and productive day**.

I knew that to run a home school would be challenging. Parag's school is an ever evolving process, so the rules get added and deleted as per need. **Discipline, time management and energy management** are also one of the major reasons why the school has been going on for eighteen years now. The main reason why there is a fast burnout rate among special education teachers is the constant, every day rigorous demand of energy, in managing the classroom and providing quality education. In taking care of special need students, energy conservation is must! The team work has worked in running Parag's school and I believe it will work in a regular school setting too. The simple logic behind this is that the teacher is relieved by another efficient teacher, so she can recharge without worrying that by taking a break, her student will regress. All these rules and decorum have been effective in the running of Parag's school.

Some concerns, issues and future plans

Parag is improving and is getting better at handling things around his life. Still there are certain things that bother me as a parent. As I have mentioned earlier, Parag does not expect harm from anyone. All he knows is to love and this makes him pure but at the same time very vulnerable. Being gullible makes him a target for social manipulation and maltreatment.

I met with a mother who has a son with autism. He lives in rehabilitation place. She told me that she was happy with the new residential place, where her son was residing presently. In the previous residential facility, he had an accident and he fractured his arm and no one knew how. The second time, in the lunch room someone hit him on the face and his two front teeth was knocked out. She removed him from that place. The big point was her son did not know how to tell her how he broke his arm. He was defenseless, when he got punched in his face. This story really made me anxious. I feel accidents happen once and the damage is permanent, no matter what, those teeth are gone forever. I am not consoled by the fact that it could have been worse!

After listening to this story, I decided to train Parag to defend himself. I started teaching him to run away when he perceives danger and take refuge behind someone he knows. I don't believe in an eye for an eye or tooth for a tooth, which after listening to the story becomes very literal. When I was a child and felt bullied, I would run and take refuge behind an adult. I taught the same to Parag. It is ironic that we teach what we know. As a child my self-defense mechanism was to run away from perceived danger and that is what I have taught Parag.

When Parag perceives danger or threat he runs away from there and finds shelter behind someone he knows. This training started at home, when Ankur and Parag got into a fight for the same toy, I would tell Parag "run come to mommy" and Parag did bolt. This extended to other children, if he felt threatened, at the day care or school he would run to the teacher. If he feels threatened by an adult Parag will go to another one. For example, if he is in the pantry and gulping sugar, which he is not supposed to, he sees me he runs to his dad. If there is no one then he will just run away from the scene of action, mostly to his room. I remember, one time Parag saw this fly buzzing and hovering over him. Parag followed it with his eyes and backed off till he was behind me. It is a funny memory because the expression on his face was of fright, it was his first encounter with a fly and he felt threatened and took refuge. Now he is not scared of flies, because many times he has seen those and we have told him that flies are okay. He is not scared of them anymore but he does not like them anyway. Who likes pestering flies? Parag won't pet other people's dogs, only the dogs he is familiar with. He won't initiate touching anything that he is not familiar with until and unless asked to.

I made him say the word "pitti," in Hindi. The actual word is "pitaie" that is beating. Pitti is a word to interact lovingly with a kid, when the threat does not have the sting! Parag knows what the word means. To teach him to express that he does not like to be treated a certain way was tricky. I would tell Parag, if he did something "bad" (bad means he is in trouble, because he has done something that is not wanted from him), I will do "pitti" (I used this word way before we decided to use English as the language spoken

143

with him), and I will tap him gently. To make something aversive or likeable is through the **voice modulation** paired with the action that made it effective and clarifies the intent of the word also. He then had to show me where I had tapped him, or done "pitti". Parag had to pair pitti with something, he did not want, so I had to enact the motion of "pitti," when he was misbehaving and had to modulate my voice as if I was upset. Once he started associating "pitti" as aversive, my job was done. Then it was even trickier to teach him to understand when, I meant it seriously and when I was using the word playfully. To teach him to distinguish, I had to choose playful moments and then use the word. He would laughingly say "no". These kinds of trainings are incidental. Therefore these kinds of training rely on the teachable moments. **Repetition is the only way to nail it down**. Parag is able to convey if he does not like being treated a certain way. When he says "pitti" that means "stop, I don't like it". When Parag does not like the interaction with someone he may also say "go away", "leave me". He does not know how to express something that happened a while ago. We are working on lessons, where he can relate to us what happened yesterday or a few hours ago. I have discussed how we are teaching this in the chapter "Teaching Communication."

Recently Parag used the word "pitti" to warn me. He had put all the lights on in the living room. I told Parag not to put on all the lights and that it was not Diwali: festival of lights. I switched off the lights. He went running and switched on all the lights back again and then turned to me and said "pitti." He was warning me as I do to him. My husband and I laughed because my teaching was backfiring on me. I have related an incident where the mother used to say "shut up" to the kid with autism. One day he used it on her but she did not like that. Well, the kid with autism must have not liked it as well and that is the word he learned from her to communicate certain emotions. So it is very important to choose to teach socially appropriate words for the children to express themselves.

Parag has limited verbal communication skills but remembers. To prove this point, I will narrate an incident. We had gone to visit our friends in Virginia. Our friend's youngest daughter and Parag were fighting for one toy, it was some kind of a wire ball that could be pulled and it became big and then it could be squeezed and it became small. She took the ball from Parag and hid it. Parag cried for it and also tried to look around, to find it. We found their altercation very amusing. That is not the end of the story. The story ends this way. When the same family came to visit us and when this girl tried to touch his toys, Parag took it away and put it back. We were so surprised that he remembered and did not want to share his toys with her.

Parag shares his things, if that person shares his /her stuff with him. For example, one of our friend's daughter's shares her chips and Cheetos with Parag. It is kind of cute to see them sitting together, watching TV and digging into a bag of chips or Cheetos. Well, when she comes to our house Parag shares his food with her. We have taught him sharing but he has taken it to a different level on his own that is to share with those who share with him. This makes me realize that he remembers but cannot communicate in words, particularly the things that have happened in the past. However, it gives me hope that he will react to people, from the way they treat him. This is a big instinct for self-preservation and survival.

Losing Parag is one of my biggest nightmares. When Parag was about six, we were at the Gulf Shores, Alabama. I realized that Parag was not in the apartment. My tummy knotted and I panicked.

I am so thankful that in times of crisis my husband keeps his cool. He asked me to breathe and took me to the balcony of the condo; he spotted Parag at the beach, enjoying the ocean. To this day I don't know how he worked the elevator, for the condo is on the seventh floor. For that matter I have not figured out how he is able to break into computer passwords and get to you tube. This was a very disturbing experience for me. Another, incident happened when he was thirteen. I was upstairs and when I came down, I could not find Parag. I started looking for him and shouting his name. My neighbor called and said that Parag was at her house. I was relieved and sank on my knees to thank God. Not finding anyone at the house, he decided to go to the neighbor's. I brought him back; I was crying and laughing at the same time. I promised to myself this will never happen again. Thankfully, seven years have passed by since and he has not attempted this again.

We had to come up with a plan of action to eliminate this behavior. It took a lot of thinking and coming up with many ideas at various levels. We got a gate put up at the end of our drive way. Cameras were put in too; this made the house more secure and a physical barrier for Parag. All the doors in the house have an electronic chime, so whenever a door is opened, it chimes. Next, we put the security system on when he is not in front of my eyes and we both are the only ones at home. Parag has an ID wrist watch, even though he knows his home address and the phone number. This is an extra precaution. This watch has his name, address, contact phone numbers and also the information that he has autism. I also think that getting a cell phone and making him carry it all the time will be a good idea, this way we can track him by the GPS system!

All the above are physical barriers put in his way but the biggest goal was to make him understand that he cannot go without letting us know. This task was daunting. I realized the above incidents had happened for two different reasons. Going to the sea shore was an impulsive need for he loves being in the water and he had been asking us and when he found that we were not listening to him, he decided to go on his own. The second incident happened because he thought he was alone in the house and he took refuge at another familiar house, in a quest to find people he knows. After the analysis, I had to chalk out a plan. First whenever he asks for anything, and we cannot attend to that right away, we tell him to wait for so many minutes and then once he has waited we make sure we give him what he has asked for. It could be giving his favorite food, to giving a car ride, etc. This applies to everyone, who is with Parag. Second, was to tell him where he can find me in the house that is in the basement, my bedroom or outside in the kitchen garden. When I leave home, I tell him I am going to do such and such errands, while these people are there. Also, everyone tells him bye, see you tomorrow or see you soon. He now understands that someone is always there in the house, he is never alone. We don't leave Parag alone. There is someone always with him. May be one day he will be able to stay at home by himself without any supervision.

At a get together, one of our friends said that we (parents) will likely die before Parag that must be a big worry for us. To this question, probability wise, the reply is "yes", but no one knows the future, I want Parag to live a very healthy and happy life. The whole system is geared towards making him as independent and self-sufficient as possible. However, I am a hopelessly hopeful parent. No one knows the future, maybe there may be some cure in twenty some years, maybe he will be able to find someone who loves him, maybe he will be so well trained by then, that he will be happy living in a group home, there are many maybes and those are the pearls of hope. To all the parents who are in the same predicament as us, I will say there are many concerns. We have and a lot of friends who occasionally play Devil's advocate. Thankfully, they give us the energy to work harder and reach for concrete solutions. I have found out from my experience that the moment concerns become worries; it dissipates the energy and does not help at all. Hope and goal oriented solutions are our best friends.

The big part of raising a kid with autism is to not worry about what might happen in future. That does not mean that you don't plan for it, actually there should always be multiple plans. If one does not work then we have another one to fall back on. The work at hand should be the focus, for it is to prepare the kid and the family to handle things better as the time goes by. To prepare does not mean to worry. I will give you an example: When Parag was diagnosed; I would worry about nth number of things, a big dissipation of energy. One of the things was how will he shave? Well, now he is there, we are teaching him and he loves the process. I guess, he sees his dad and brother shave and when his turn came he was ready for it. I used to envision it as something Parag will dislike and we will have a hard time teaching him this skill. In my mind, I would visualize him throwing tantrums and injuring himself with the razor. I would be terrified with the thought of it. **The lesson learned is: Do not let your imagination run haywire and see dreary things in the mind's eye.** If energy is channeled, to the task at hand then the results are discernible. What is to happen is not in our hands but to prepare without worrying makes life more fun. It is important to enjoy the journey. When I look around, I feel we have come a long way. So my concerns are genuine but they are no more worries.

We have created an environment where Parag interacts with people who care for him. As a parent it is very hard to know that your child can be taken advantage of and he/she may not be able to defend themselves and seek the right help or communicate about it. In spite of all the training I have described, Parag is still vulnerable. He does not expect harm from anyone. This makes me very protective of Parag. We have surrounded him with people we trust and who love him very dearly.

Puberty

When Parag hit puberty, I had a new set of questions. I know by now that getting professional help is not only wise but a very quick way to alleviate confusion. It is a shortcut to gain knowledge from other peoples' experiences and repertoire of knowledge. I set up an appointment with Parag's pediatric neurologist, for I knew he would point me in the right direction. I asked him a question that was bothering me a lot, Parag had started touching himself and I wanted to know how to approach this. He laughed because he perceived my discomfort and said that I should approach it the same way as I do other things for him. He said that Parag does not know some appropriate social behaviors and he will learn those if coached. He smiled and calmly said that there is nothing wrong with Parag, his hormones are kicking in and he is acting normal, it was me who was reacting abnormal. He also tried to console me, by saying that as Parag grows older his urge will plateau.

He also brought up the subject of Parag moving in to a group home when we are too old to take care of him. I was so stunned and the thought of not having him with me tore my heart. My husband had often tried to talk about this but I wouldn't listen. Coming from the pediatric neurologist's mouth was even worse for I had to listen and swallow it whether I liked it or not. Talk about bitter pill! As a post thought, I think it was good that he reiterated what my husband was trying to tell me. He also said to take tour of various facilities and then decide which suits Parag's needs and if we are comfortable with him being there. He let me know there was a big waiting list in these places so it is better to apply and if we did not need it then it will roll over but we will be made aware of the vacancy. He did suggest a few places as well.

I came back very pensive for it is hard to be brave all the time. The fact that I had to train Parag to not touch himself in public, a social taboo, was a challenging task and on top of it the very thought of ever parting with him, not seeing his mischievous smile everyday was unbearable. I am still not ready to see him live away from me; it is a heart wrenching sensation to just think about it. Maybe the reason is that I don't think he is equipped enough for that life style yet. The fact that Parag in many ways cannot defend himself and can be taken advantage of is a predicament in itself. In spite of my trepidations and anxiety I decided to check out a residential facility, I have described that in the chapter "Visit to the residential facility."

I had to plan how to make Parag understand that touching himself in front of people was not appropriate. If he has the need to touch himself, he has to go to his bedroom, his private space. The training has been successful for he now realizes that he needs to be alone in his room. This training was same as making him wear a towel after a shower. He did not care, for nudity is again a social taboo and I had to teach Parag that he needs to wrap the towel around himself.

When Parag was about four, we went to Orange beach. I put Parag in the swimming pool and I went in the shade, under the gazebo, to read a book. In a few minutes some little girls came running to me, huffing and puffing and said that my son was skinny dipping! I bolted and asked Parag to come out of the pool, holding a towel to wrap him in. Parag swam to the deeper end; I had to get in the pool to get him. Everyone was laughing at the commotion and I was the only serious one in the lot. Now I am able to laugh at the incident, at that time it was not a joking matter. This incident made me, teach Parag to wrap himself in a towel the moment he stepped out of the shower. Parag is not ashamed or shy when he is naked. These are learned social behavior and now he wraps the towel around him because he has been conditioned to do so.

When the house is full of boys then coaching certain appropriate social behaviors are very difficult. Ankur tells me that if I allowed it, Parag could win the burping championship, for Ankur has trained him well. I stopped Parag's tutelage of burping by Ankur at infancy. Parag still imitates his brother and burps! I don't allow this game but I have a suspicion that the brothers play this game behind by back, just a mother's hunch!

The hard part about training for appropriate social behaviors is not that it is any different from other behavioral conditioning but the fact that we perceive a lot of social taboos with shame. I was distressed because sex and masturbation were subjects that were never openly discussed while I was growing up; it was a socially taboo subject. This made me anxious because I perceived Parag's behavior of touching himself as shameful. After talking to Parag's pediatric neurologist I realized that it was my thinking that was creating anxiety. I also thought that I should be happy that my son was maturing into adulthood normally! Once I was able to fix my thinking and see no shame in Parag's action, I was able to teach him how to deal with his needs and desires, so that it is socially acceptable.

Conditioning of Parag's Behaviors

We teach Parag by applying Applied Behavioral Analysis previously called behavior modification. Conditioning of behaviors is a big part of Applied Behavioral Analysis. There are certain aspects to well-rounded teaching that need emphasis and elaboration through the perspective of conditioning of behaviors. There are certain subtleties and extrapolations that go beyond the theories. When we apply behavioral conditioning many variables comes into play in real life situations. Theories are proved under controlled environments. Real life situations are dynamic and ever changing.

Before I talk about some behavioral conditioning that we have done with Parag. I will clarify my point. I want my readers to know about two renowned psychologists in the fields of Behaviorism, Ivan Pavlov, a Russian scientist and B.F Skinner, an American psychologist. You must be familiar with Pavlov's dogs experiment. The dogs in this experiment started salivating in response to the sound of a bell (neutral stimulus) which was repeatedly paired with the presentation of food (unconditioned stimulus). After a few trials the dogs started to salivate (unconditioned response/reflex) just with the sound of the bell. They started associating the sound of the bell with food. This response of salivating with the sound of the bell was learned, this was now a conditioned response. This is called **classical conditioning. Simply put salivating in response to food is an inbuilt reflex, an involuntary response that does not need learning but when salivation occurs with the sound of the bell it is a learned behavior.**

B.F Skinner came up with conditioning of voluntary behavior by using either reinforcer or punishment. In this way a desired voluntary behavior can be strengthened or weakened. Skinner is known as the Father of Operant Conditioning. **What is an operant? It is a response. Simply put the whole theory is how to get desirable responses**

Skinner put a hungry rat in a Skinner box. The box had a lever on the side and as the rat moved around, it accidentally knocked the lever, and food fell. The rat soon learned to go straight to the lever and press it to get food, the reinforcement. Moreover, it learned to do this again and again, that is the frequency of this behavior increased.

In the next experiment he introduced an electric current, an unpleasant stimuli, which gave the rat discomfort. The electric current would stop once the rat pressed the lever. The rat learned to go straight to the lever. This way it escaped the pain by pressing the lever and this is called escape learning. The next variation to the experiment was that Skinner introduced light just before the electric current was introduced to the box. The rat learned to press the lever the moment the light was switched on, thus he learned to avoid the painful experience of getting an electric shock altogether. This is called avoidance learning.

What is the basic difference between Classical conditioning and Operant conditioning? Classical conditioning involves the association between involuntary response/reflex and a stimulus. Operant conditioning focuses on associating voluntary response and consequences. Also Operant conditioning believes in reinforcers but classical conditioning does not. Classical conditioning requires no active participation from the learner because it stimulates a response that is hard wired in our system, like salivation. However, Operant Conditioning requires learners to actively participate and perform a task in order to get the reinforcement or the punishment.

What is common between Classical Conditioning and Operant Conditioning? Both types of conditioning lead to a change of behavior which facilitated **learning**! This is exactly what I wanted to happen for Parag: learning. I have related the experiments purposely because with my experience in training Parag, I have realized that these theories are not as compartmentalized as in their experiments. When I started teaching Parag through applied behavioral conditioning all these theories got amalgamated and got me results. The conditioning of Parag's behavior and learning of skills took place by combining these theories into practice. I have found out that practical is different from theory. Theory gives the overall idea for handling things; it could be a behavior or learning a new skill. When it comes to a real life situation combined with mind boggling Autism Spectrum Disorder, believe me all these theories have to be customized for every single child with autism. Applied Behavioral Analysis heavily relies on techniques of behavior modifications with special needs students. These are some of the behaviors we have been able to modify by using both the above techniques in a unique way.

When Parag was three, he used to walk on his toes. I have described in the chapter: Early intervention: Teaching life skills, daily Living Skills and getting rid of some Symptomatic Behaviors. I have stated in that chapter that I made Parag wear shoes with hard sole, so it would be hard for him to walk on his toes. In this case I had to eliminate a behavior. I also believe that Parag was not doing this purposely, he was not even aware of this. So it was an involuntary occurrence. I wanted him to become aware of it and stop walking on his toes altogether. When he tried to walk on his toes particularly when he was not wearing the shoes, I clapped or clicked my fingers and pointed at his toes and said "heel down" and physically made him plant his heel on the floor, so that he could understand what was asked of him. I then let him walk. I praised him for doing so. Gradually, he connected the clapping to not walking on the toes. He became aware both of his toe walking and that he should not do it. Then, I made him look in my eyes and pointed at his toes and he would stop walking on his toes. After that, all I did was look in his eyes and he would stop walking on the toes. Initially the noise, the clap and the click were necessary because the sound got his immediate attention, once he was aware pointing was a better option, but silent communication through eyes is best. The reason is that clap and click will draw unnecessary attention of people when out in a public place. **I believe behavioral teaching should eventually become as subtle as possible and only the teacher and the student should be aware of the learning taking place.** After all social camouflaging and social acceptance are one of the main goals for all children with autism. I have used the same technique with Parag for hand flicking also. The moment he flicked his hands, I would clap or click my fingers and then asked him to put his hands in his pants pocket. Once he became aware of hand flicking, which he was previously unaware of, then all I had to do was look in his eyes and point and he would immediately put his hands in his pockets. The next phase was to just look at him and then he put his hands in the pockets. Putting his hands in the pockets is a coping skill along with a camouflaging of a behavior that otherwise draws unnecessary public attention. The concept is the same as Parag wearing hard sole shoes, it made it harder for Parag to walk on his toes and camouflages the behavior. In the case of hand flicking putting his hand in the pockets makes it harder for him to flick his hands and camouflaged the behavior. Parag looks cool when he walks with his hands in the pockets! We praised every successful trial, gradually he did not need any praise for this. Parag does not walk on the toes anymore, so this behavior is extinguished. He occasionally flicks his hands and a lot of times puts his hands in his pockets before it occurs, so this is a behavior that lies dormant and then it comes back, now we have to look in his eyes and he knows what to do! I believe by making Parag put his hands in his pockets and also making him walk in a hard soled shoes restricted the expression of the sensory behaviors of flicking his hands and walking on his toes respectively. This lead to the subduing of hand flicking and elimination of his toe walking. Logical analysis is that the brain did not get the desired unrestricted responses for the signals that it was sending to these body parts. Over time these signals were not strong, due to the behavioral interventions, so these behaviors subdued both in intensity and in frequency.

I cannot definitely put these conditioning of behaviors as classical or operant conditioning. The reason is that these behaviors are due to sensory stimulations, therefore involuntary and this falls in the category of classical conditioning. I praised Parag for every successful trial in the beginning, so this makes it operant conditioning. To extinguish behavior generally unpleasant stimuli is needed, as with rats in the Skinners experiments. Well I did not use that either. Once these behaviors were extinguished and generalized both stimuli (pointing) and the praise (the reinforcer) were faded or they were not needed. **I am a firm believer that aversive/punishments of any kind will extinguish a behavior but cause a lot of behavioral altercations between the teacher and the student.** As it is, there are so many issues that need to be addressed when dealing with autism. Why make one more by making the student irritable, when he should be pleasantly complying.

I have trained Parag not to open the door for strangers. This behavior modification was very challenging because Parag was opening the door for anybody and everybody. The moment he heard the doorbell he would go to the door and open it. Once someone rang the bell, I would follow Parag and make him look at the person. Our front door has a wrought iron design with glass on it. When he looked at the person, I would say "stranger, don't open door, go inside" and made him go back. If it was someone who was coming to the house often, like his play buddies or the teacher, then I would say "friend, open door." I purposely used short phrases, to keep the communication simple. I did emphasize and reiterate the words "stranger" and "friend." He needed to understand that he needs to open the door for friends only. When Parag did not open the door for people he was not familiar with. I would praise him by saying, "good not opening the door for a stranger". Gradually he was able to distinguish between people for whom he should and he should not open the door. He will not open the door for UPS or FedEx delivery men. This does not mean that he is not curious about the parcel they bring. The moment I retrieve it, Parag wants to look inside and see if it is of interest him. Anyone who comes to repair something in the house, electrician and plumber are also strangers to him, because he does not see them often and they are not familiar to him.

The funny thing is that Parag is now thinking of who is a friend and who is not. Parag opens the door for his caregivers, family and discriminates between our friends too. Our close friends, whom he sees often, also the ones who acknowledge him and interact with him; he classifies them as his friend and opens the door for them.

Our friends who don't visit the home often or friends who don't interact with him, Parag does not open the door for them, they are strangers to him.

Recently, he opened the door for Ankur's teacher. She has been coming for some time, and she acknowledges Parag and also brings amazing desserts for us. One day when she rang the bell, Parag went to the door, looked at her and after few minutes of pondering and hesitation opened the door for her. She and I laughed because that day he put her on the list of his friends. I think this is what he thought at that point in time. She has been coming here often, she is nice to me, brings me stuff, so she is my friend, I should open the door for her! So you have to be Parag's friend, not just ours, for him to open the door for you!

I believe that conditioning is something that we do to each other all the time. We react a certain way because of certain inputs (social, verbal, physical, emotional) and the reaction is the behavioral outcome. When a child throws tantrums to get a toy in a toy store and he/she gets it, then the person who bought that toy conditioned a behavior. There is the likelihood that the child will use the same behavior of throwing a tantrum to get something else. If this goes on for a while then it is a learned behavior from the situation or the environment. Many times, we parents are guilty of reinforcing an inappropriate behavior and then when it gets out of hand we blame the child for it. It is not the child who is to blame! We all as parents teachers and caregivers need to think about the consequence of the conditioning of a behavior and then intervene with a plan.

Dr. Watson and Rayner wanted to prove that the reaction of young children "crying" when they heard a loud noise was prompted by fear. Through classical conditioning they wanted to show that an unconditioned response, a reflex like fear could be associated to another stimulus that a child would not fear normally. To prove their hypothesis they found an emotionally stable nine month old child "Little Albert." I always think of him as "poor Albert". These psychologists exposed Little Albert to various stimuli, including a white rat. The baby showed no reaction, a neutral stimuli and he was allowed to play with it. Then they paired his interaction with white rat with loud noise. The moment little Albert tried to touch the rat or tried to interact with it, these scientists made loud noises behind his back by hitting an iron rod with a hammer. The baby would start crying. After repeated exposure he started crying by just seeing the white rat. The pairing of the loud noise was not required for he was scared of the white rat. The scientists were able to prove their hypothesis; learning did take place through conditioning of a behavior. Little Albert also showed stimulus generalization, he was fearful of Rayner's fur coat and Watson's Santa Claus beard. That is he transferred his learning to other similar looking objects! What did he learn? He had a phobia or extreme fear of furry things? Without the behavioral conditioning he would not have been fearful of these objects. I don't understand why it was necessary to mess up a normal child's brain? As a mother to a special needs child and as a special education teacher, I spend my time in rectifying and conditioning Parag's brain to become as normal as possible. **The reason I have related this experiment is that it is our duty as parents, teachers and caregivers to think and analyze the long term effects that may happen to a person whose behavior we are trying to condition. It is a matter of great responsibility!**

For example, "Time-Out" is a behavioral intervention in which the student is placed in a less reinforcing environment for displaying certain behaviors, such as tantrums, aggression and being off-task. However, in the case of children with autism this could be overtly reinforcing. Many children with autism like to be left alone and Time-Out is what they want. If the frequency of misbehavior increases after time out and gradually misbehaviors become more vigorous, then the teacher should rethink her intervention. Time-Out is not working.

A mother of a child with autism told me that she used to send her child to his room whenever he misbehaved. I asked her if that had stopped him from misbehaving? She said that actually he was misbehaving more often. I asked her to find out what triggered those undesirable behaviors, and if it was task avoidance then make sure she stuck to her guns because it felt like he was misbehaving to go to his room. This advice was right out of the top of my head because there was a time when Parag misbehaved while doing a task and I would send him to the corner as Time-Out. He started throwing tantrums even more and I started sending him to the corner even more. What made me ponder was when he went in the corner the behavior evaporated and he would just stand there quite still. My "eureka" moments have been through observations of Parag's behaviors. I realized that he was misbehaving because going to the corner was exactly what he wanted instead of doing the task at hand. Sending Parag to the corner as Time-Out was actually reinforcing his behavior to get out of the task. Once this was clear to me, I brought about the real conditioning of this behavior. When Parag threw a tantrum to avoid a task, I would increase it. I would also tell him why I was increasing his work load. I would tell him "Parag is a bad boy, so he will have to work more." Once he understood the consequences of his task avoidance, he straightened up his act. He definitely did not want to do more work. However, the transition to the desirable behavior to make Parag perform the task was hard because then I had to make him do it, even when it took me hours. The reason it became harder was that through Time-Out I had already conditioned his behavior and then I was trying to undo a conditioned behavior or a learned behavior. To undo a conditioned behavior and replace it with a new one is a difficult task. All this leads to a major war of will between the student and the teacher. **So, it is very important to define a problem and figure out concrete behavioral modification plan because once it is a conditioned response or a learned behavior it is very hard to change it.**

I also have related that Parag used to shoot out of my sight like an arrow and he had no fear of being lost. In the chapter: Early interventions: Teaching life skills, I have described how we trained him to be with us and not leave his caregivers. To check on his fear of being lost all I would do is take him in a public place with many people, like the mall and when he seemed to be engaged in seeing something and not aware of my presence, I would hide where I could still see him. Within a few minutes, he would become aware that I was not around; Parag would not only start looking for me, wide eyed and also sometimes he started crying. So when there are many people around him in a public place, he holds my hand or the hand of the caregivers. Otherwise, he walks with his hands in his pockets, which we have taught as well. However, when Parag thinks that there is a possibility of getting lost, that the place is too crowded with people, he will hold my hand tight, which I don't mind; after all we have conditioned him thus.

As I have said, before conditioning a behavior we should consider a lot of scenarios and then see if overall this is a beneficial behavioral conditioning. I have stated in chapter: "Exercise", that Pranav and I have started running races with Parag. Guess what? Parag holds on to my hand while running. We are the only people in the race who are doing tandem running while holding hands! There are many people in the race and Parag does not want to be lost. Parag is hyped up and happy before the race but once everybody starts running he perceives confusion; hence his reflex of getting lost is triggered. I believe after a couple of runs he will feel safe and realize that we will be running with him, so he does not have to hold hands. Of course I have to talk to him while I am running, like: "Parag is safe, everyone is running without holding hands, Parag can do that to." There are many mini talks going on when Parag and I are running; most of them are encouragements. Pranav too goes on bucking up Parag while running "Come on Parag, you are doing great," or "Come on, we are almost there." Gradually, I will have to see if he will leave my hand for few seconds and then go on increasing the time until he does not hold my hand at all while we are running. This is a process and if we go on making Parag run races, the repetition of the stimuli will generate the conditioned response of not holding hands while running. Parag will **figure out** that it is safe to not hold hands while running. We still run together but without holding hands.

I have stated in the chapter: "Behavioral interventions that have worked for Parag," that he used to sometimes run away from his classroom and come downstairs. I did put locks on the classroom doors but I did not want him to learn in a locked environment. It was a temporary coping skill for the teachers, a physical barrier. I had to plan an intervention process and behavioral conditioning, to overcome this situation. I asked the teachers to **never** physically force him into going back to the classroom; it could lead to injury to Parag or to the teacher. Teaching and learning has to be an amicable process and forcing Parag to learn could have led to aversion towards learning. I asked everyone in the house to hide, and then asked the teacher to ring the front door bell, while I hid too. Parag looked for everyone and not finding them went to the door and opened it for his teacher and went back to the classroom. Now if ever he runs from the classroom, which is rare, the teacher has to ring the front door bell, all we need to do is tell him "go open the door," and he does that and goes back to the classroom with his teacher. **Behavioral conditioning is a powerful tool.**

Conditioning can also lead to "learned helplessness." In simple terms, learned helplessness is when a person starts thinking there is no point in trying. Many times, special needs students think they will be unsuccessful with a particular task or skill, so there is no point of trying and they give up. In the case of Parag it is different. He is not depressed, he is happy and knows how to wrap us around his fingers and get things done for himself. Parag's learned helplessness has come from the fact that he is able to manipulate people to do things for him. He does not do something because he will get another person to do that task for him. When Parag was about four years old I taught him to say "help me." When he said that I would be thrilled to help him with whatever he was doing. I thought that this was a great thing I had taught Parag because he will be able to ask for help when he needs it. Little did I know that he would start using this phrase with his charm and make other people do things for him? Both Parag and the person who helped him, felt good for different reasons. Parag was happy because he did not have to do the task and the person who helped him felt good because they felt gratified and satisfied in helping a kid with autism. Parag also hugs and kisses his caregivers for helping him and of course smiles all the time so lovingly. It took me time but I figured out that he was making us his slaves through his charm!

I had to muster a strict resolution not to fall into the trap of helping him. The moment he asked help for a thing he was able to do, I started saying "no, you help yourself," for things like drying himself with the towel, dressing himself. There were times he would say "give me please" and believe me the word "please" pleased me so much that I used to give him whatever he was asking for. The reason I was happy was because verbal communication is something we teach Parag. He was using language to communicate, so I felt so thrilled that I would do stuff for him like a person who is mesmerized. Once I was able to see that by doing things for him I was making him more dependent on us. The goal was to make him as independent as possible. We were conditioning him to not perform the task that he was very much capable of doing on his own. I gradually stopped helping him or caught myself before the urge! So after this realization, when Parag asked "give me please," I would say "take it yourself." These were chores like giving him water, pouring juice for him, warming his food in the microwave. Parag did not like me for not doing his work but he soon realized that the rules had changed. Parag also tried to seek another person, to do things for him, thinking that my mom is not doing this for me, but others may still do all these things. He was wrong; everyone was on the same page. Parag realized if he does not do his task then no one else would do it for him, so he might as well do it himself. Sometimes we leave the room after telling him that we cannot help him and that he has to help himself. With no one around, he is forced to work for himself.

During the early phases of the homeschool, when Parag was doing his worksheets and he made a mistake, I would erase it for him and then he corrected his mistake. One day, when he made a mistake, I said, "no wrong, fix it." Parag turned around the pencil so that the eraser was facing towards the paper and then handed it to me. It was a very illuminating moment. I had taught him to be dependent on me by erasing for him whenever he needed. Parag had not spoken a word but silently he had communicated volumes. From that moment onwards I stopped erasing for him. **This incident seems benign but is utterly serious. The reason is, we make our children dependent on us, we condition their behavior of "learned helplessness" and the scary part is we are not even aware of this.** This incident made me pause and self-analyze. The answer to the musings was that I was in a hurry to make Parag finish his worksheets and that made me develop a habit of doing things for him along with the erasing his mistakes on the work sheet!

Patience is the name of the game! No matter how much in hurry I am, I have to slow down and let Parag do his task himself. There were times when we had to go somewhere and Parag was not ready, I helped him to get ready. When we have to go somewhere and we are running late, I have a natural desire to get Parag ready and get going. Parag as intelligent as he is, figured out that this was another way to not do what he is able to do because when mom is in hurry she will do it for me. It took a lot of control and patience to not help him and make myself think that being late to an appointment or an event is not the end of the world. Both Pranav and I are very punctual and to be otherwise bothers us. I know Parag is smart and to outsmart him takes planning and thinking. A couple of times I left him at home when he was not ready, he did not like that because going out and being with people is something he likes very much. So he realized that if he does not get ready in time, he would miss the party!

It takes immense patience and time to uncondition a learned behavior and learned helplessness is no different. The only way to mitigate and extinguish this behavior is by not helping, when that person does not require help. As teachers, parents and caregivers, it helps if we make a list of things with which we are helping the children with special needs when they don't need it. After a while a list is not necessary but in the beginning it helped to see how many things I was doing for Parag that I did not need to do. It was a great feeling to scratch out the tasks and skills from that list as I stopped helping Parag and he started doing those things on his own. It is encouraging to children when we tell them they are very able and capable to help themselves. This re-in forces their independent work and performance. This also bolsters their self-confidence.

Parag still tries his tactics of learned helplessness around people whom he knows will do it for him. For example, when his grandmother is here, he will stick his socks in her hand and ask her to put the socks on his feet. I have tried to tell his grandmother not to do it but her reasoning is that she is not with Parag all the time and since she just visits us once in a while, doing what he is asking for is all right. This is an emotional trap, and I have given in to this thought process, thinking she is getting old and this is her way of having that special bond with her grandson, so let it be. I have realized that in running Parag's homeschool, I have to respect loved one's emotions too and cannot make every teaching process cut and dried or clinical. The repercussion is that when grandmother is around and we don't do a task for Parag, he goes to her. This means that he is **discriminating between people** who will and who won't do things for him.

Lots of things do not need conditioning of any kind because Parag learns from his environment. For example, Parag loves to swim in the pool; he is a fish all summer long but during September when the water in the pool gets cold Parag dips his feet in the water and comes back inside the house. He perceives the change in temperature biologically. During the winter season, Parag stands on various air vents all around the house, because he loves to warm himself with the warm air coming out of the vent. During summer when he gets too hot, Parag takes showers. Another thing he does on his own is waiting for his caregivers. Once he is getting ready in the morning for his school, he looks through the curtain for his teacher's car. In the afternoon, he waits for his play buddy to come and play with him. He often goes to the front door and looks out for their cars. If you ask him "Parag are you waiting for your friend?" Parag will say "yes" or "yes waiting" or "yes I am waiting for" and he will name his friend as well. The talking part has been taught incidentally, while he is waiting **but no one has taught him to wait** for the people who are part of his daily life. I have stated in the chapter: "Decision to speak in English around Parag," Parag uses Hindi words and phrases appropriately and in the right context. Thus some learning took place by sheer osmosis of observation and hearing. This is definitely not a part of these conditioning processes.

Parag has learned a lot of things just by observations and perception of his surroundings. He expands his learning through generalization and applies his schema to new situations and tries to problem solve as stated in the Chapter: At what level is Parag functioning? Parag thinks for himself and makes a decision (cognition and metacognition).He is also discriminating between people to see who will fall for his trap of helping him, so that he can avoid doing work by himself. **We explain the reasons for the teaching of skills and tasks.** We talk to Parag and he understands why we are asking him to do and not do certain things. Explaining and talking is certainly not a part of classical or operant conditioning.

The point is that these theories are very helpful in understanding and modifying behaviors but they are incomplete. A person's environment does modify his behavior but there are other factors that also influence how we behave. Such as genetics, neurological connections, information processing: thinking, problem solving. Using schema or applying prior knowledge to a new situation are also factors and variables that come into play in real life situations. We need to analyze, synthesize, expand and extrapolate these variables in applying behavior modifications or intervention plans.

Power of reinforcers

The dictionary definition of a reinforcer is "a stimulus, such as a reward, the removal of an unpleasant event, or a punishment, that in operant conditioning maintains or strengthens a desired response." **Never underestimate the power of reinforcers.** We all need reinforcers of some kind. That is, we need a pat on the back once in a while to feel appreciated and encouraged for what we do. The reinforcers, like praise from the boss at work or at home praise for fixing a good meal makes us not only feel good but to try even harder. It is the biggest motivator for all of us. It is the same with children and even more so for children with special needs. I have seen it work wonders not only with Parag but with any student. Before we can use any kind of reinforcers we have to believe that special needs children are capable and that they can learn. Then we have to encourage them to their highest potential. A high expectation is a belief system that every teacher, parent and caregiver must have to make the children with special needs blossom.

I had the privilege of teaching a girl who was in fifth grade but was working at a second grade level. I volunteered my time two days a week and one and a half hours each day. First day I just talked with her, tried to gauge her feelings and fears. I told her that I was thirsty and that I wanted her to show me the vending machine. I offered her a soda as well, this turned out to be an icebreaker, for while drinking our soda we talked. She told me that she did not want to study because she was stupid and that everyone in her class teased her. It was sad to see her weep, while she related how she felt. She said that she did not have friends and that she hated school. I told her that I related to her feelings of not having friends, and told her my story. She was very still and all ears while I told her my story. I told her that until third grade I did not have friends and like her, I used to eat lunch alone. This all changed for me when, one day my class teacher, Ms. John asked everyone to name their friends. I said I had none, she said that was not true because she was my friend. During lunch time she asked me to come in to the classroom, where along with her children I started eating lunch. During the lunch time Ms. John would tell us amazing stories, some of them I remember still. She taught songs and made us sing. Once I graduated from her class, I started making friends on my own. **She had taught me the biggest lesson in life, if you want something then reach out for it.** After telling her my story, I said that I was there to help her just the way Ms. John had helped me. She agreed to work with me because a relationship of trust was created between us, a great start.

I knew the biggest problem with her was she had very low expectations of herself. I had to make her think that she was capable. Just like teaching Parag, I started with edible and tangible reinforcers pairing it with praises and encouragements for every baby step towards the desired direction. Eventually, compliments became her biggest reinforcer, just like Parag. Meanwhile, her work improved. I found out that her parents were not educated and could not help her with homework when she got stuck. I gradually directed her to ask for help from her teachers. As her grades improved, her desire to do better increased. Success is very intoxicating and for the first time she was experiencing it, gradually she was becoming competitive. She also started believing that she was bright, because by the end of the sixth month, she was working at fifth grade level. This is one of my best experiences as a teacher.

The point I am trying to make through this experience is that **motivation is one of the biggest reinforcers**.

Choosing right reinforcers is very important. The student should want it, so he/she is willing to put in work to get it. In Parag's case, we started with edible reinforcers, like cookies, candies, coke and tangible reinforcers like twirling objects, top, pin wheel, spinning disco light, a massager, and television shows of his choice and songs/ video clips on the i-Pad. These are tangible reinforcers and are also called primary reinforcers. We paired praises and encouragements with his entire task along with these reinforcers. During the early phases of the homeschool, tangible reinforcers were used a lot. I felt it was cumbersome and many a times we would be off schedule. Managing time and being on schedule with all the breaks and primary re-inforcers was challenging. I felt that it hindered the tempo of teaching and fast pace learning. I believe these were necessary to increase his compliance during the initial phases of the training. However, Parag, narcissist that he is, soon learned to love praises and compliments. After all, reinforcers are something the student likes and to get it he works harder. Pairing praises and compliments with the primary reinforcers and then fading away the primary reinforcers made teaching him easier and our time could be managed more efficiently. Fading away primary reinforcers does not mean that we do not use it at all but it means that we use it less and that Parag is not dependent on those to perform a task.

The above are examples of positive reinforcers, giving something desirable to the student on completion of a task. The negative reinforcers work well too. The word negative attached to the reinforcer makes people think negative reinforcer is something undesirable and that students don't want those. On the contrary, students love negative reinforcers. If a teacher tell the students that if they maintain a ninety percent and above, that is grade "A," then that student will not have to take the finals. If this incentive of not taking the final exam motivates the students to work harder and perform better, then the negative-taking away something, is really reinforcing. The reason I am elaborating this concept is because one time I was in an awkward situation for using this word. I was talking to a parent as how she can use both positive and negative reinforcers to gain compliance in her child's work. She got very upset, thinking that negative reinforcer meant punishment. I tried to explain but the word "negative" had ticked her off.

Negative reinforcers have nothing negative about them! Simply stated, it means removing something, that the student does not desire or want, and this leads to favorable and desirable outcomes. For example, one time Parag did not want to write, and he was telling me I want to go downstairs (the classroom is upstairs). I told him you could go, if you write down what you are saying. He wrote: "I want to go downstars." I let him go. I was amazed that he could almost write downstairs without teaching that word. So by letting him go, I got a desirable behavior of extra effort of thinking on Parag's part. When Parag does not want to do a certain worksheet, then I make him do just half but he has to do so quietly and without misbehaving. The concept is simple. I scratch your back and you do the same for me. So as a teacher if I am making your task less demanding by cutting it in half, which is what you desire, and it makes you feel less ruffled, then you make my life easier by behaving properly and not throwing a tantrum, that makes my life less ruffled too. Another criterion is if there are twenty questions in the worksheet and Parag is challenged by those, then we may ask him to do ten questions, and come up with seven correct answers. This way he can concentrate on performing better than trying to finish a worksheet to get over it without even trying. If he is able to do this then he can leave the rest of the questions. So by decreasing the task I am able to get better performance and less misbehavior, then surely the negative reinforcer has worked. I want the readers to know that negative reinforcers have nothing to do with punishment.

As I said above, we should choose the reinforcers judiciously. Parag used to love staring at the credit cards and I used old credit cards that were not active as a reinforcer. He used to stare at the numbers and the emblem. Well, I learned my lesson in a funny way. I had invited some friends over to my house. The next day my phone started ringing like crazy, my friend started calling and telling me that instead of their credit card, they had another friend's card in their purse.

I realized what had happened, Parag had taken everyone's credit cards out from their purses and after playing with them, technically staring to his fill, he put them back, but not in the right purses. Well, I apologized and explained what had happened to all my friends. Now we laugh at that incident, but I learned an important lesson, never use things of value as reinforcers. So things like a check book, expensive jewelry (for some autistic children are fascinated with shiny jewelry) and of course never use a credit card as a reinforcer! Reinforcers are powerful but we don't need to make them expensive, for then they become a liability.

I never thought that a reinforcer could become anything more than a thing to make student comply and want to perform their tasks better. Parag has proven me wrong. Parag loves balloons; we used these as a reinforcer, during the early phase of the school. Blowing balloons at my niece's birthday party, we all were busy decorating and Parag started blowing and tying all the balloons, he is as efficient as a balloon pump or may be even more efficient! This gave us a great idea, when our friends are throwing a party and they need balloons to decorate, then Parag comes in real handy and a big help in the decoration process. **I had never imagined that a reinforcer could become a useful skill!**

Punishment is something we need to talk about in this context. Punishment is some kind of aversive that is used to mitigate or diminish an undesirable behavior. **I believe that punishment works at a very high cost.** It may lead to more behavior problems than necessary. The reason is many times children with special needs are not motivated to perform their tasks and to avoid that they are ready to misbehave and then punishment such as detention works as a reinforcer because getting out of work is what they want. Punishment may lead to desirable behavior eventually but with a lot of unnecessary altercations between the teacher and the student. It becomes a battle of will with parties, the teacher and the student thinking "let me show you." Sometimes punishment makes the special needs children even more hardened in their undesirable behaviors, a way to demonstrate a silent rebellion. Silent rebellion is very powerful. Instead of complying and cooperating they become totally immune to the punishments.

Let me clarify this point through a movement in India during British rule. Mahatma Gandhi had started a non-cooperation movement in India, where people showed their grievances against the British Empire. Indians stopped cooperating with the British rule non-violently or peacefully in spite of the punishments. The result was British had to give India its freedom from their imperialistic rule. I totally believe in finding a peaceful and amicable solution to a problem. After all coming from India, I want to embrace and practice Mahatma Gandhi's philosophy of non-violence. **I don't believe in punishment.**

Having a bad feeling, losing energy on enacting a punishment is not very practical. Punishment brings about anger and resentment in the parties, the student and the teacher. There are chances that a student can retaliate with aggression towards the teacher or towards himself. It is also possible that the teacher can be unduly aggressive to the student in his/her state of anger.

The children and especially the special needs children should think that teachers, parents and caregivers are on their side. By punishing them we make them think otherwise and there are chances they will start thinking of us as their enemies instead of well-wishers.

We have to find the reasons behind their misbehaviors or undesirable behaviors, and then we can plan a behavioral intervention that is more sensible. I believe in creating discipline and talking to the student. The first and foremost thing is that we have to believe that the children with special needs understand, therefore talking to them is of utmost importance. Parag is limited in his expressive language but receptively he understands just about everything. I have seen that when I talk to him and explain why he should not do something or why he should do something, this gets me the desirable responses from him. In the case of children with autism there are certain sensory behaviors that needs frequent reminders. Explaining to them the reason to control those behaviors not only makes them aware of their involuntary behaviors but lets them start applying the coping skills taught to them.

In my experience, I have noticed that we don't talk to children with autism, we deliver commands and expect delivery or enactment of those commands. This is a very robotic and mechanical interaction. The unpleasant situations or misbehaviors occur less if communication channels are open. Communicating our needs and feelings is also re-inforcing in itself. Through teaching Parag, I have seen that by talking to him, and **warning/reminding** him to straighten up his act leads to desirable behaviors. Praising him for being good makes him want to be good. This is surely a better course for both of us then throwing down a gauntlet.

Sometimes **ignoring** an undesirable behavior works too, particularly when the whole drama is put on for us. It is easy for me to do this with just one student, Parag. It is more challenging for the teachers with many students. Another thing is to have **rules and consequences.** This way there is no surprise element for both the teacher and the student. **The Student knows what is going to happen and the teachers know what to do if the rule is broken.** In my classroom the rule is simple.

- Rule: Parag is going to be a good boy. (Parag knows being a good boy means to comply and co-operate with the teacher)
- Consequences: When Parag is a bad boy, he will not have breaks. (Parag knows being bad in the classroom means losing his most favorite reinforcer and those are breaks between the transitions from one subject to other).

We don't have many rules in our classroom so it will be less confusing for Parag. We are able to verbally enforce this because of its simplicity. Before we enact our consequences we warn/remind him of what is going to happen if he does not get his act together. Parag is praised for being good and not praised for being bad and he is reminded why the breaks are being taken away. The sentence is simple "You are being bad so you cannot have the next break." We never take away all the breaks or the reinforcers from Parag. Removal of all the reinforcers takes away the motivation to work and leads to behavior problems. The thought process is why put forth an effort when there are no rewards?

Reinforcers are the most powerful tools for a teacher. In teaching Parag I have found out the biggest reinforcer I have is **voice modulation**. When I praise him, he knows it is praise because my voice is full of enthusiasm and when I am not happy because he is doing something he is not supposed to, I have to use my firm voice. I know its effectiveness through using those to bring compliance and motivation in Parag for his tasks. **As with any powerful tool, reinforcers have to be used judiciously to produce fast and successful results.**

Visit to residential facility

I made an appointment to visit a residential facility for adults with developmental disabilities. This took a lot of thinking and finding courage because checking out this place meant that I was now preparing myself to the idea that Parag may one day be able to fit in there, if the need arises. Pranav and Parag's pediatric neurologist had talked to me and asked me to be open to the idea of phasing Parag into a residential facility which was a good fit for him. The logic they proposed was that a time will come when we may not be able to take care of him because of old age or some unforeseen turn of events. I conceded for one reason and that was to satisfy my curiosity about the functioning and care that is given in the residential facility.

My husband, Parag's teacher and I went to check out the residential facility. I was totally blown away by the founder of this place, a simple hearted farmer, who started this place some twenty years ago, for he could not find anything to his satisfaction for his special needs son. He came up with the idea of a safe and caring place for individuals with special needs. He gave his land and dedicated hard work to create this non-profit organization. To see that this place has emerged from a personal need for love and care for his own son in to giving the same to others who needed it too, was heartwarming. I was very pleased to see that the homes were well kept and every home has a supervisor to oversee its smooth functioning.

There is a vocational training center, which provides meaningful, productive employment. I got to see the workshop where many individuals were doing different activities. Some were putting some car parts from various trays into a zip lock. About 4 to 6 individuals were in a group and a job coach oversaw that everything was going smoothly. What impressed me was that all the individuals were sitting down and doing their work very diligently. They also have a huge green house and many residents grow seasonal flowers which they sell. The best thing is they enjoy the process and also earn pocket money. There is a special building for individuals who need twenty four hour care. The impressive thing was everyone was clean and looked well taken care of. It was an eye opening experience for me because I did not expect this efficient level of care! I was humbled because I just take care of my special needs son. Here there were caregivers who were dedicating there love and time to special needs individuals, who were bed ridden or in wheel chairs. Some needed help and assistance with everything. I felt tremendous respect for the caregivers and could not fathom their magnanimous hearts!

I came back with a lot of positive feedback. I also realized that to be able to function efficiently in this setting, daily living skills had to be mastered as much as possible. Parag's curriculum has become more structured towards daily living skills since then. He has to make his own bed, take out the dishes from the dish washer and lay the table for dinner. He cleans up his classroom and art and craft area and vacuums and wipes his desk with Lysol towels. He brings the trash down stairs and dumps it in the big trash can. Right now all this is monitored by the teacher. Once it is time to clean up, she reminds him and goes on asking "what do you do next," to see if he can remember the sequence of the chore. She may just stand there and see if he will do things without prompts. Gradually chores will be added as he masters these. I realized that chipping in to the household chores has to be done by every member of the family, but for Parag this is a survival skill. The funny thing is he thinks taking out the dishes from the dish washer is a game. We had taught sorting to Parag from a very young age. We used to put different things in front of him and would ask him to "put with the same." This skill was taught by using the real things and through flash cards. For example, we used to pile up the cutlery and then make him sort those and stack them in the cutlery tray. We also piled clothes in front of him and he had to sort them in the same category- that is pants with pants, shirts with shirts. We haven't done the sorting of clothes with colors, but once we are ready to tackle laundry skills, that will be yet another skill for him to learn. This skill of sorting has come in handy and the practical example is emptying the dish washer and then stacking them away. The first day we showed him where all the utensils are and then modeled how to do the chore at the same time saying "put with the same." He connected and knew what was being asked of him because he has sorted things into various categories in the classroom. What was totally unexpected and pleasantly surprising was that Parag also likes doing this chore. I have absolutely no complaints! Parag has learned to make his bed and set the table for dinner. He is becoming a big help around the house. I see that many skills that have been taught in the classroom setting have transferred into Parag's daily life and sorting and organizing things is one of them.

I believe this skill of sorting can help children with special needs to become efficient in their daily living skills and also help them to find jobs. For example: sorting cutlery in restaurants, filing according to alphabetical order. The avenues are numerous and teaching sorting needs to be explored with the job aspect in mind. The very fact that the special needs individuals at the residential facility were sorting car parts into a zip lock for a Honda car plant is an encouraging example of employment due to sorting skill.

I am so glad that I visited the residential facility. This has reduced my anxiety that if Parag goes to a residential facility he will not be taken care of. What I have learned from this visit is that I have to equip him with all the skills to succeed in living in a group home.

Vocational training

After the visit at the Residential facility, I was thinking of involving Parag in some meaningful vocation, that he can enjoy. I started racking my brain, what could Parag do, at his skill level and interest. We went to the local Rehabilitation center, and they recommended an evaluation for Parag. He went with his teacher for the evaluation. The evaluation stated that Parag could not be trained for any job at this point in time. After reading the evaluation I was heartbroken and started crying and praying to God for guidance. The Lord has mysterious ways!

While I was crying and praying a voice spoke in my head, "It is October (2012), Christmas is round the corner, why don't you teach Parag to make candles, people love candles". I was thrilled with this idea, with zero knowledge of how to make candles, I went to Hobby Lobby and got a book on candle making and supplies too. I had to learn the skill, perfect the glitches, break it down to easy steps and then teach him. **I knew that I could not teach him the experiments but only the results.** Parag will emulate things as taught and it becomes very hard to make him unlearn or to change it. Even before I could teach him to make wax candles, I decided to stop, for it was too dangerous for Parag. The double boiler system of heating up the wax is cumbersome and then the moment wax falls on the stove, it catches fire. I went on researching and to my delight found information about gel candles. I was pleased to know that gel is made of natural ingredients such as 95% food grade mineral oil and 5% resin, a plant product. It is more luminescent and burns longer than wax candles. Due to its transparency, it can be versatile and if it did not come out right, it can be reheated and poured again. **I needed a craft that was forgiving of mistakes.** This all sounded perfect for my next experiment.

I bombed with so many candles that I have lost count of them and found that when gel fell on the stove, there were fumes and I read that these fumes are non-carcinogenic. I wanted Parag to use the stove as little as possible, so I got a presto pot for melting the gel, with temperature settings, it is perfect and I also asked my handyman to attach a faucet, so that Parag could collect the melted gel in a container.

Once I was ready to test the ones I thought had come out perfect, they were not so perfect after all. Once I lit them, the wick drowned in the gel. Then after researching a lot, I found out, that the local store keeps low density gel and the wicks are not at par with the quality I was seeking. **This was not a craft project but a vocational training.** Thus quality mattered a lot. After researching, I ordered high density gel and the right wick attached to the zinc sustainer base, so there was no chance for the wick to float in the gel. **The best thing that has happened is that Parag enjoys the learning process.** I was quite taken aback by the speed at which he could wick and cut them with precision too. Pouring was easy for him, for he has good hand-eye coordination. The tricky part was to teach him how to add color and how much color to add. The same goes with the fragrance. Weighing all the raw material on the scale was cumbersome. I wanted to keep everything simple, so I decided we will use volume measure for making the products. So the measure is in cups and spoons, which works like a charm.

After removing all the glitches, Parag made around eighty candles for Christmas gifts. This really gave him good practice. After

Christmas, once we had given most of the candles as gifts, I realized he wouldn't be able to make more until next Christmas. I said this to one of my friend's, who had a gift shop. She asked me to show them to her, to my great surprise, she said she could sell them. Her endorsement and vision that Parag's craft was something people would buy has kept his vocational training an ongoing process. This initial support helped Parag to go on making his candles. People love Parag's candles and write heart touching comments of encouragement for him. Moreover, through his candles, his story is spreading, showing that kids with autism are capable. All they need is someone to show them the path and believe in them.

Learning is a continuous process, so Parag's candles are getting better with practice. He started with making beverage candles. The first candle he mastered was a coke candle. The reason was simple, black color did not require precise measurements. He is learning the finer techniques, such as how to have bubbles in the champagne candles and not to have those in the martini candles. **The beauty of the process is that we are learning together.**

The real artist in Parag got a chance when he started making pottery candles. Parag loves to paint and he won't miss a spot. He is totally absorbed and happy creating his art and painting his pottery. This is a much more involved process. The first step to making these is to roll the clay and then put it in the mold. Well, Parag was not able to roll evenly with the rolling pin. I got the tortilla maker and now Parag presses the clay in it and the clay is perfectly even. In special education, we always talk about improvisation and assistive technology to enhance productivity and skills. This is an example along with the example of using a presto pot with a faucet for gel melting for the candles. **From my experience of teaching Parag, I have realized there are always many possible solutions to a**

problem. Road blocks are there to make us sharper and if we cannot climb over the road block, then we can circumvent it and still be on the desired path. It may take longer, but the student will reach the destination. After all it is brainstorming to the nth degree. There has to be a solution, there is a solution! All I do when I face a road block while teaching Parag is go on thinking and brainstorming with the team and then there is always an "aha" moment.

One thing I did in the beginning was to teach Parag to make candles through verbal instructions and a lot of encouragement. The process had a concrete result and Parag was able to see his efforts take shape into these beautiful candles. The same way I taught him to make soaps. Parag uses his soaps and sees his candles lit at home. This must have given him the reason to make them along with the fact that he simply enjoys making them. Now we read the recipes and then make the products. The concept is similar to teaching reading to young kids, first they have "learn to read" and then "read to learn". We inculcate enthusiasm towards reading by first reading to young kids, so they understand that these letters when together make words and sentences which make these stories! They have to see the bigger picture to want to learn to read! So I first immersed Parag into making crafts, so it had meaning to him. Now we are learning the nuances of creation by breaking it down into steps. He now reads the recipes and follows the directions. What I see, as I teach him to make all these products that we are using his knowledge in a practical application. Parag is counting and measuring while making the products and all that makes more sense than just doing worksheets. I believe it crystallizes his learning from the classroom to the work shop, our garage and basement! Parag's enthusiasm to learn is making him become more independent.

Every product that has come about has a story and has been made due to a personal need. I could not find products that are pure, natural and without chemical preservatives in the market. What propelled me to research and then come up with my own recipes is Parag and I have very sensitive skin and we have allergic reactions to many products. One time Parag broke out with rashes after taking shower, it was the shower gel that caused those rashes. I decided to make our own soaps with no chemicals and preservatives. After experimenting with those, I realized that these soaps were gentle to our skin and safe for sensitive skin. This gave birth to the next project. That was to teach Parag to make organic soaps. We grow loofah in our kitchen garden. Parag gets to water the plants, pluck the gourd, clean them, cut them and then embed them in the soap. That is how he makes loofah soaps. I like these involved processes for him, because they are not monotonous and give variety to the craft, while he is learning. People liked the soaps. I realized that there are people who would like to try simple, pure, organic products. The fact is when people read the ingredients on the labels of the products of PM Candles; they are familiar with those ingredients and are willing to try it without hesitation. To keep the product simple and with few ingredients also helps in teaching Parag. I give the products for trials to my close friends and some pharmacists; they use it and then give me their input. In this way we are able to tweak it and improve it. In the winter I made the first batch of the lip balm because Parag and I have chapped, dry lips during this season. I did not want to use petroleum jelly lip balms and the ones which were supposedly organic had too many chemicals and preservatives in it. So I researched and came up with beeswax lip balm with honey in it. Well, the first batch had too much honey in it. The input I got was: we love it but it is sweet and we love to lick our lips. I already knew this because Parag would put lip balm on his lips and lick it away. I knew I had created a dessert instead of a lip balm. I experimented again with my recipe for lip balm and came to a balance, where it is not too sweet and has the right consistency. I also figured out how to make honey mix well with the coconut oil without it sinking to the bottom of the container because of it is of higher density than the oil. **Once it was approved by my "testers" I started teaching the recipe to Parag and the whole process of labeling and packaging. The teaching process is rigorous but the fact that Parag is an enthusiastic learner makes the whole process worthwhile and fun!**

Last winter Parag had nummular eczema. The treatment is to moisturize the skin. Thus came about the organic body lotion with sandalwood rose essential oil. This summer my yoga teacher asked me if we were making any natural bug repellant. Parag has allergic reactions to bug bites, so I cover him in bug repellant before he goes outside or in the pool. I was aghast to read all the chemicals that these bug repellants have particularly- **DEET** (N,N-diethyl-m-toluamide), which can be very detrimental for mental and physical health. I came up with a natural bug repellant which has combination of neem, basil and citronella in coconut oil base and vitamin E. Thus this organic product came about organically thorough a conversation! We know that bug repellant is effective because it got tested by lots of families and kids on this fourth of July.

Initially, I came up with recipes where Parag made things with ten cups of oils . Well, he fell in love with number ten. So when he was filling the spiced heat pad with spices, he wanted to fill ten spoons of spice mix in the bag. I tried to tell him that he just needed five but he did not pay attention and went on filling the bag . Once the bag got overfilled and the stuff started falling out he gave the bag to me . I showed him that 5 spoons full was enough and after that he just emulated and corrected himself. When Parag was not doing right, I did not stop him because I wanted him to see that this was not going to work and once he saw that, Parag was ready to learn the right way. **The lesson from this incident is everyone has the right to make mistakes and learn from it. In teaching kids with special needs we are so bent upon getting the correct responses and reinforcing them that we don't give them the chance to make mistakes and learn from it.**

One of our close friends made a website for Parag and my husband, who is passionate about photography, took pictures of Parag's crafts. The website is: www.pmcandles.com and I like the video section, for people get to see Parag working and learning. Since this is a project, we don't sell Parag's products through this site, they can be bought at two stores and a spa in Gadsden and they also ship the product if there is such an order. Their endorsement and support has given Parag a chance to improve on his crafts. The gratification that these products are of value and are selling is re-inforcing to teachers involved in Parag's life. All of us feel proud that people like his creativity. When there are orders through these stores, we all get so hyped up and have a peacock syndrome for a while. Parag just loves making these candles, soaps, creams and balms; he does not understand the value of money, so he can give away all his candles and soaps for a bag of chips, one of his favorite foods. He loves the process of creating, that the product he makes is of some value is not his concern; all he wants to do is make them.

I hope this vocation can turn into a **steady source of income** for Parag. I feel that as a parent, it would be an immense satisfaction for me to see that he can financially sustain his upkeep. That means affording the salaries of his caregivers, his own needs (clothes, food etc.) and to be also able to treat his friends with ice-cream and movies! I do have a dream that one day he will have a shop, where we can display not only his crafts but crafts made by other special needs individuals. Everyone should enjoy the dignity of labor. As promoter of Parag's craft and spokesperson, I have realized that his craft has to evolve and he has to go on making something new and different to appeal to the people. The product has to be high quality and unique. **To come up with new ideas is always a dynamic process but it is even more challenging when I have to think at Parag's skill level, to simplify it and break it down. So that he is successful in reproducing the products and it is fun for us.** This takes a lot of experiments and we are the biggest consumer of our experiments. I see that anytime we come up with a new product or when just improving the old ones there is a lot of wastage and that is not cost effective. This process not only requires patience and perseverance but money as well. I foresee that any project of this kind won't sustain itself until and unless it breaks even and ultimately earns a profit. We have been able to sustain this because Parag's happy, focused energy in making these craft gives us hope and zeal to go on.

To spread Parag's story, we also donate for various causes and have started giving out products to fund raisers. The Student Council for Exceptional Children at Jacksonville State University, does fund raisers with PM Candles, this not only gives us the opportunity to sell the products and spread Parag's story but it also gives us an opportunity to help other special needs students. Parag has found enthusiastic support from ladies at Yoga class in Anniston. They are our best clients because they believe in organic, "go green" ideas and Parag's products fit in perfect with this mindset. I want Parag to have a client base who believe in pure, simple handmade products that have no artificial preservatives and harsh chemicals. He makes these with love, just like a home cooked hearty meal!

I did not know that the guiding voice "in my head" was initiating me on a journey which started with candles and now it has diversified to so many other things. Parag's story inspires many people; his story shows them that special needs individuals are capable. **All they need is someone to show them the path and believe in them.** I believe every parent should look into their child's potential and scaffold them to learn a satisfying hobby and vocation. It is heartwarming to read all the encouraging comments people write to Parag, in the comment book at the shops. I am going to share some of those with the readers; they will be attached at the end of the book. I cannot think of a better way to culminate this journey. The best wishes from people who believe!

Why is Parag happy and what has worked for us?

How do we know that Parag is happy? Parag always smiles when he interacts with people and laughs too. This is a very outward manifestation of the inner feelings. His laughter is so infectious that, no matter how hard the day has been, it brings a smile to everyone face. Is he happy because he is content with himself and his basic needs are met? Is he happy because he is not on the wild horses of ambition and hoarding of material wealth? Parag reminds me of laughing Buddha, a pure soul, who loves everyone and unconditionally. Everyone he is surrounded with loves him too but our love has not transcended conditions like his. **This is a big part of Parag's happiness to love and be loved.** Apart from this metaphysical aspect of explaining why Parag is happy, there are many concrete reasons.

The reason he is happy is he gets treated at his emotional or mental age. He is still a kid at heart, and to treat him at his physical age brings a discrepancy between his physical age and his mental age. If he is not there biologically, then he will not understand and not understanding will lead to behavioral escalations. Gradual, stepping up in our response to his growing up mentally is also very important so we change the interaction accordingly. For example- when he was young, he would love to snuggle between me and my husband, and would resist sleeping alone on some nights. Now, for a long time, he developed a need for his own space and loves to sleep in his own bed. It happened mostly naturally but we went on letting him know that "Parag is a big kid, he needs to sleep in his own bed." Parag used to sit on our lap till he was six, we told him that Parag was a big kid and he needs to sit on the chair, gradually he stopped sitting on our laps. The point is, you do go on saying and doing what is expected but it also happens naturally when the child is developmentally ready.

Parag likes to watch musicals like Mama Mia, Disney movies and Barney. Parag watches SEC football games with us. He enjoys movies in general but the fast paced movies particularly the car chase ones, are his favorite, like Fast and Furious, Need for Speed. What a thrill seeker! Backstreet Boys is his all-time favorite. Right now he loves listening to Lady Gaga's album; I know it will change after a while. Parag also listens to Hindi songs. He navigates on his I-Pad, pulls up the songs he wants to listen or the movie videos he wants to watch. Someone asked me to stop letting him watch Barney and the Disney movies, because he will never grow out of it. He is still a kid at heart! The fact that it does not bother me is I don't find it wrong or inappropriate. I still enjoy the cartoons that I watched when I was a kid, like Tom and Jerry, Donald Duck and Mickey Mouse. It makes me laugh and makes me nostalgic. Parag too has the right to choose what he wants to watch and hear. This is a big part of our individuality. I believe he perceives all the children in Barney as his friends; he has grown up watching them and also loves the songs. As far as Disney movies are concerned, I am a big fan of Disney movies, great entertainment, with awesome messages to mankind. Actually, I love to watch these with Parag. Parag has ear for music, he also picks the songs from watching these movies and sings to himself. It is very entertaining when he sings "Love will find a way... and Can you feel the love tonight.." songs from Lion King. I wish everyone had a kid in them and have the ability to just enjoy! Parag is happy also because he is able to enjoy his choice of movies and songs.

Parag is happy because his school changes with his changing needs. We understand that one of our biggest requirements is to enhance his interests. He is given a chance to show that he is able and capable in his own way. School accepts him as he is and then creates opportunities to enhance his innate abilities. Expectations are high and directed totally towards his abilities to shine. The teaching process involves an amalgam of visual, auditory and kin-esthetic inputs, so that it is as concrete as possible. Parag learns and understands better if things are presented to him in a concrete manner rather than abstractly.

The goals that are set for him are realistic and achievable by filling all the gaps. This makes Parag successful. It is a huge gratification to the teachers and caregivers. "Nothing succeeds like success." It gives everyone the zeal to continue. The goals are not just set by a report card, our way of Individualized Education Plan. I also make New Year's resolutions for Parag and myself. I have found out that if I make resolutions for Parag, then I am not only more vigilant for his success but also for the success of my resolutions. One of the resolutions this year was to make Parag lose weight and he has lost about sixty pounds. In making Parag eat healthy and follow an active life style we all are doing the same. These achievements make Parag more functional and make him a happier person.

Early intervention has worked for Parag. Early on it is vital to chart out a plan, short term and long term, to work on the major deficit areas: **communication, social skills and behavior problems.** Initially, I along with the team, worked on mitigating the symptomatic behaviors of Autism. I felt the less of those the more social camouflaging and social acceptance is possible. Increasing communication also helps in increasing the quality of life of the autistic child and the family. If a person is well behaved and pleasant, then he or she is not only accepted but also liked and people want to interact with them. The same goes for the individuals with autism. Parag is always well dressed, happy and smiling, which makes him approachable.

Parag has developed good hygiene habits along with proper grooming which works for us and makes him more acceptable socially. Kids with autism deal with many challenges on a daily basis and it is better to avoid any sickness. Hygiene is directly related to good health. It is better for kids with autism to learn personal hygiene and keep their surroundings clean. When any one is well groomed and clean they are more socially acceptable. The same goes for children with autism. I like Parag to be properly dressed when he goes out. This also lets him blend in with the norm. Of course, he has an advantage, for he is handsome too. I know all of you reading the book must be thinking, well that is a mother's thing. Every mother thinks of their children as handsome and pretty. I have related that Parag is a narcissist and he has become so because where ever he goes people say "You are so handsome". This has definitely gone to his head, for he loves to admire himself in the mirror and if you ask him "are you handsome," he will say "yes" without any humility! Parag is friendly, loving and well groomed, so all this leads to his social acceptance, and that makes him happy as well.

Coping skills for the behavior problems have worked for Parag. Everyone has a need to vent their emotions when they are frustrated and upset the same goes for the kids with autism. As a teacher and caregiver we need to teach them appropriate social responses to a behavior. For example, Parag starts to bite his wrist when he is frustrated, so we give him a hanky to transfer his need to bite, this way he does not harm himself. He asks for a break before he gets too frustrated. Coping skills are a learned behavior and a necessary tool for functioning.

Parag is happy because he is an active participating member in our family. Parag does not feel left out as a family member and is able to go everywhere with us, to restaurants, movies, games and vacations. **The biggest part of his inclusion is that we talk to him and he responds back.** If we take a person everywhere with us and still do not talk to them then it is not inclusion in the real sense. Parag knows that he is not only included in all that the family is doing but he is an active participant. Parag is able to reach out to people and get their love and affection. This naturally makes him happy. Parag has been able to learn and also is included in many social activities because of his ability to sit and enjoy. A lot of our learning sessions require sitting down for some time. When we go to the movies, games, shows and restaurants, we have to sit for a considerable amount of time. If the kid with autism is not able to sit for a while, then it is very difficult for the parents and caregivers to take them to these activities. For Parag sitting down properly in the classroom was generalized to other settings because we took him with us to all these places that gave him the opportunity to demonstrate his skill of sitting properly in real life situations and settings. There were times when Pranav and I took turns and ate in the restaurant. Parag was either misbehaving or refusing to sit. We still took him with us because he had to learn to behave properly in that context. The fact that we are able to include Parag in vacations and are able to take him to restaurants and movies has worked out both for Parag and us.

Creating and customizing a program that is meaningful in the real sense has also worked. We want to see Parag grow into a wholesome person, with likeable qualities. For example, he looks into a person's eye, smiles and replies to the overtures. **It is a pleasure to see happy Parag and all the skills and vocabulary that he has, to use for his benefit and with comprehension.** He is able to generalize on his own and this is a boon, for I have seen many cases where this does-not happen even after modeling and coaching. The life skills and daily living skills have helped Parag to become gradually more independent and the process is ongoing. The more independent he is, the better it is for him and his caregivers. Caregivers have one less task to do for him! Eventually, a system has evolved that works for Parag and our family. He needed more one on one and a personalized schedule, which worked with his pace and was an enjoyable process for both the teacher and the student. To move on slow and steady is better than move fast and crash! I have always believed in the tortoise and hare story. **In this competitive fast paced world, to slow down and gather focused energy, for the children with autism at their learning pace is crucial.** Home school was what we chose. For, I foresaw a happier Parag and family.

Another, thing that has worked for us, is that Parag follows directions. This makes life so easy and the training to make him follow instructions was not just for worksheets and tasks in the classroom but in the real setting. By following the instructions Parag has become more independent in his surroundings and also he is able to help us. All this training required repeated modeling and demonstrating what we were asking him to do. For example, if we have to go somewhere, we ask Parag to change his clothes and be ready, which he very willingly does because he loves going out. If we ask him to go and turn off the lights in the room or close the door, he does it. Parag has learned to listen to verbal commands and understand non-verbal cues. If we do not want him to behave a certain way, we let him know. The ultimate warning is if he misbehaves, we will take him home. Parag, as I have mentioned earlier is a party animal, he loves to be where all the action is going on, so the warning to take him home is a big one it straightens him out. He also knows that we mean what we are saying. It has happened in the past. He has been taken back home and we repeatedly told him why we had to bring him back home. The sentence generally is "Parag was a bad boy". "You were misbehaving, you were bad, so we brought you back home." Over the years, Parag has figured out that word "bad" means he is in trouble and he should not be "bad". Now we seldom have to use the verbal warnings. What we still do is non-verbal cues. For example, he may be fiddling with the straw for his drink and all we have to do is look straight in his eyes and shake our head in a gesture "no." Or just look at him and make a facial expression as if we do not like what he is doing, he reads that expression and stops.

Having a supportive and understanding team has been an asset; this has kept the school chugging along. Over the years many teachers have contributed to how Parag is today. Everyone has chipped in, and contributed in their unique way. Having a team breaks the monotony, having more than one teacher brings variety, because every teacher has their way to impart the same skill. The team gives everyone time to recuperate and rearm new strategies for road blocks. It also gives an opportunity for the teachers to learn from each other and go on with more fortitude. Parag's buddies, who come in the afternoon to play with him are also teachers, difference is they teach incidentally and many things are planned, so it is not accidental. This interaction is informal versus the morning sessions.

Gardening has been such a pleasurable activity for Parag and me. I think a great hobby for children with autism is gardening, where a lot of teaching happens automatically. It helps lot of children to desensitize with their tactile/kinesthetic issues, like touching dirt. Plucking, homegrown organic vegetables are one of Parag's and my most pleasurable activity. There are immense teaching opportunities in this activity. This has given Parag the opportunity to identify various vegetables that we grow. While we are harvesting these, we can incidentally learn so many things, nothing like learning colors through plucking off various colored bell peppers, tomatoes, egg plants, chilies, beans. There are times watering the plants turn into a water day, both of us are wet and happy. Ultimate pleasure is when we make salad and sandwiches from the fresh harvest!

We have found some common activities that all the family members can do together. Ever since Parag ran his first 5k, we have decided to make this our family activity. Parag has an exercise regimen; he walks on the treadmill for one hour every day. I believe this not only keeps him fit but also helps him to sleep well. He is hyper, so exercising, riding a bike and playing badminton, ping pong or swimming makes him tired and helps him sleep well.

The most important thing is the **mindset** that makes things work. In Parag's case, the whole family has joined hands to help not just Parag but each other as well. The therapist and Parag's buddies do not work for us, they work with Parag. All of us are a team with unified purpose. To us, to make Parag as functional as possible is the goal. To reach this goal, we are trying to create a system that emanates harmony and balance for all of us.

Epilogue

This book is about our journey to tackle autism. Autism does not have a cure. It also is a spectrum disorder which makes it very ambiguous to deal with. There is no single right approach because every individual with autism has their extraordinary challenges. Every parent I have met is fighting their own battle of autism in a unique way. Our story is yet another unique story. **Through this book I want to convey to people dealing with autism that we are all together in this journey: Our journey.** This book is not focused on details of teaching techniques. The intervention plans and teaching methods have just helped to convey the story. It would be great if any of those help parents and caregivers. Finding the right direction when someone is groping in the dark is a way out from the tunnel.

To deal with Parag's autism, we choose a new path. The whole idea was to not only help Parag but to bring a balance and normalcy to our family. This does not mean that the system we have created for Parag and us is better. It is a great satisfaction that the approach is working for us. Parag's intervention plan has not been focused on academic success but the three deficit areas that are challenging to the children with autism in general: **behavior problems, social interactions and communication.** The homeschool is geared towards making him more functional and socially acceptable. When stereotypical behaviors along with asocial behaviors are reduced, the social acceptance increases by default. I have also seen that social acceptance for children with autism, actually for all children' increases if they are well groomed and well dressed. We work to increase Parag's communication skills which is our main teaching objective these days. We also focus on making him more independent around his daily surroundings. All the efforts are to see him burgeon into a happy, wholesome person, in spite of his challenges.

Through our story, I want everyone to see, that eliminating confusion and then deciding what we really want for our child with autism is essential. Clarity of thought is an absolute necessity to execute any idea. This helps channel the energy in the direction we are striving for. I wanted to have a life as normal as possible, in spite of Parag's autism. We decided to have the back up of a research based approach: Applied Behavioral Analysis, under which all these teaching styles fall: Incidental teaching, Discreet Trial Training, Contextual Teaching and Teachable moments. Along with these techniques we use a common sense approach with a lot of patience and love. We want Parag to be as independent as possible. We have tried to bring this about by amalgamating various teaching styles and trying to avoid falling into the trap of teaching Parag "learned helplessness." Finding right re-inforcers, now mostly praises have been a boon in teaching skills and conditioning behaviors.

The first thing to help kids with autism is to build a strong family with clear views on how to help each other along with the kid with autism. The tips and anecdotes are helpful for caregivers to create a balance. We had to create this system because the public school system was not working for Parag but this system of home schooling clicked with him. The fact that Parag is happy makes me believe that many other kids with autism can also be contented through application of this holistic approach.

Before we can incorporate all these teaching modes and approaches, we have to create an environment which is conducive to meaningful learning. At home the parents and caregivers should have high expectations for the kid with autism and at school the same goes for teachers. However, to make the student learn, he /she has to be motivated. The student should find the lessons meaningful. This is very hard with kids with autism; they don't understand why they are learning certain things. Many times teachers try to fill in the gaps, so they can reach the target skill. I find it easier to teach Parag, when I explain why we are learning a particular skill. For example, Parag is willing to revise his vocabulary and take spelling test, if I let him know that it will be easy for him to read the story. Most of the time he chooses a story, he wants to read. The simple logic behind this is, if he chooses he is more motivated to finish it. I have seen the magic of re-inforcers through teaching Parag and other kids. Even when they find a task hard, they are willing to perform it for enticing reinforcers! All this is possible when the environment is conducive to learning and most of the behavior problems have been sorted out through behavioral interventions. **So the elimination and reduction of behaviors during early intervention is a boon! I believe the early intervention, teaching life skills, daily Living Skills and getting rid of symptomatic behavior is a stepping stone towards actual learning to take place.**

Early intervention is must! This has been proven by research and I am witness to its effectiveness through Parag's improvement. My publisher had many questions regarding this book but the one question which I want to share is —**"Can you explain how your book could be applicable to those with children suffering extreme forms of autism who may be unresponsive?"** My response was- " When a child has autism, no matter how severe, early intervention helps tremendously. You have heard a "stitch in time saves nine"; well it is totally true in the case of autism. The only way the kid with autism becomes unresponsive and wants to be left alone, is when intervention is done too late and they are too deeply set in their ways. To bring them out of their cocoon is unimaginably hard and a lot of times caregivers lose hope. They may not respond well to an intervention approach that is not well planned, is not done consistently and persistently. From my experience I know that early intervention is a Herculean task and once that is overcome, kids with autism succeed and show tremendous improvement. **The biggest hump is the right early intervention and reducing and eliminating symptomatic behaviors and giving them coping skills for behaviors. The answer to your question is after doing all this there is no way the kid with autism will not show improvement. They can if we believe so.**

I know it is very hard not to worry, when one has to take care of a special needs child. It is a grueling task to take care of them day in and day out. I believe, if we can turn these worries into concerns and take a practical approach then many solutions become discernable to the otherwise fuzzy mind. In the book I have related how I used to worry about the day Parag will have to shave. Well, when the time came it was not a problem at all. Looking back I feel that I could have utilized that time more effectively in dealing with the task at hand with Parag. I made myself unhappy thinking of something that could happen in the future. No one knows what the future holds but to ruin the present because of that is not very productive.

I believe while teaching kids with autism it is essential to slow down and laugh. When Parag does something silly or funny I am able to see and laugh with him. Teaching and learning then becomes a pleasurable activity. You have heard "laughter is the best medicine." It is cathartic and energizing. In taking care of a kid with autism life becomes scheduled and somewhat serious. To really help the kids and ourselves we need to pause sometimes and look around us to see the progress that the child with autism has made, this is the greatest reward for caregivers. William Henry Davies has beautifully said that by worrying and not slowing down we are missing out on the beauty that surrounds us "What is this life if, full of care. We have no time to stand and stare…A poor life this if, full of care. We have no time to stand and stare."

I also feel that sometimes when we chose a path and a belief system, it may not please everyone and we may be subjected to criticism and curiosity. Autism is such a mindboggling enigma that if I was not convinced that my choice of dealing with it was right for us, I could not be here with a happy ,inquisitive Parag! After choosing a path, working hard and diligently, has also been my choice. My grandma's story helped me deal with criticism very effectively and I want to share with my readers.

There was a very talented artist, who made a masterpiece. He kept it at town hall and asked the people to mark anything that they did not like about the painting. When he came back to get the painting , he was dismayed to see that entire painting was marked, there was no spot unmarked. He was disheartened and told his wife that he will never paint again. The wife knew that he loved painting and that it was his passion. She asked him to put the painting back in the town hall and again ask the people to correct what they had marked and did not like about the painting. This time when he went to collect it ,no one had corrected anything. He told his wife what had happened, she smiled and said " your painting is perfect ,it is easy for people to find faults but very hard to fix those." Basically my instinct, conviction and education has guided me that Autism: Our journey and Finding Happiness is the path for us.

It is never easy to deal with a chronic disorder like autism but the **mindset** makes it less hard. Actually, it has given us the wisdom to enjoy small successes occurring in our lives. For us, the way to conquer autism is to work diligently and regularly with Parag but also enjoy the process itself and include the near and dears in his progress. We grab and make opportunities to have fun while treading this road of Autism. With this approach, we have found harmony and ultimately happiness. I believe to conquer anything, including autism while enjoying the process is a real conquest!

Peoples' comment on Parag's crafts and the You-tube link

It is said that "seeing is believing," so this link will clarify many things that I have written because you will be able to see somewhat linear progression Parag's progress. This also enables the readers to connect with the story, get to know Parag and his family. I also hope that it will encourage parents and caregivers.

I feel that peoples' comment for Parag's crafts are a very befitting ending to this book. Their comments have not only warmed our hearts but also gave us tremendous encouragement. I want to convey to each and every one of them, that we are thankful for their support it has kept us going. This has given me hope not just for Parag but for other special needs children. I feel they all have unique skills, which can be turned into meaningful vocations. All they need is someone to believe in them and show them how to bring out their skills to the world. People are there to appreciate it and encourage them in their journey!

Please go to you-tube link :Autism Our Journey and Finding Happiness. Readers can see videos of Parag performing various activities, interactions with people and happily making his crafts. I wish these videos will make parents, caregivers and teachers hopelessly hopeful!

12/15/12
Parag, this is just an amazing project. We would love to see you do more & more. Thank you for giving such a wonderful gift to the world as you are such a great one too.
Wanda Camei

Parag we are very proud of you. The candles are amazing and so beautiful. Love you.
Rau Saachati

Dear Parag,

Mrs Trin is so proud of you! I miss you so much. Keep up the good work! You have came such a long way. I am so blessed to be a part in your life.

Love MRS TRIN

Dear Parag and Family,
Hard work is paying off that is why we never stop
Love MA. David & Family

The candles smell amazing!

Kuryn Patterson

Parag,

I have just been introduced to your products. I used the lip balm, the hand cream, and the foot cream last night. I am amazed how soft my skin feels today. Thank you for making these wonderful products.

Martha Merrill

Parag,

I love your soap! It is so relaxing at the end of a long day. I can't wait to burn your candles. They are going to make my house smell wonderful.

Love,
Tracy Windle

Parag,

The soap smells wonderful. Can't wait to give it a try. Thank you.

Glenda

Hello Parag,

I love your products!

Tracy

Parag,

U am buying a second round of creams and soap Love it all!!
Martha Merriel

Dear Parag, & Mamta

Thank you so much for providing such a wonderfully clean line of products! It's so nice to recognize each ingredient. They make my skin feel & smell beautiful! The candles are great, too.

I would also like to thank you for allowing me to showcase your products. I am honored to be a link to such an amazing and uplifting success story!

Your Friend,
Toni McCord

I have been using the face mask for several weeks, and I love the effect it is having on my skin. Thank you!! Toni used the attar & it was great!

Ellie Field

I have the face mask and I love it!
I feel like it gives me a beautiful glow :)
It tightens & smooths & I swear it gets
rid of crows feet. Love love love it!
augr Gregg

I love everything. The lotions
are fabulous!! Mad with the candles!
Love it all? Amy M. Mauwsa

Thank you so much for the soap,
candle and pottery. The scents are
inviting, the pottery is great, and
you know how I love orange
and blue! Your talents are
shining through your work.
May your work and story continue
to touch others.
Love,
Laura McCarty

Dr. Beard:

I am glad to highly recommend this book "Autism: Our Journey and Finding Happiness" to all families, friends and educators who have an interest in working with students with autism. In this text, the author describes, in detail, the trials and successes of their journey by working together to find a way to become happy with life and find a vocation that is rewarding both economically and emotionally.

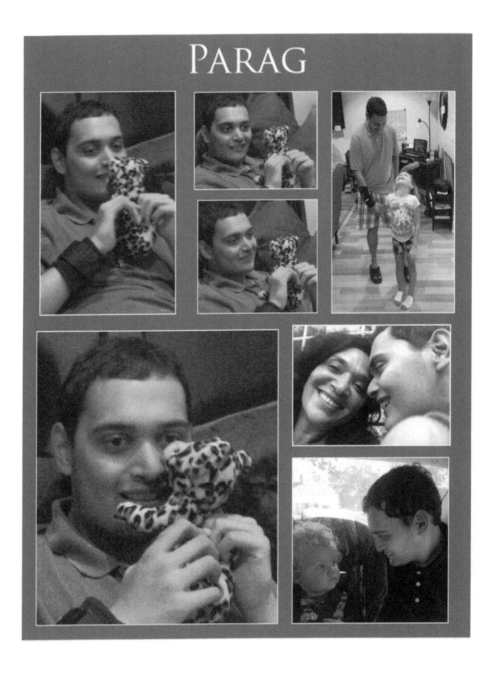

PARAG

Mamta Mishra

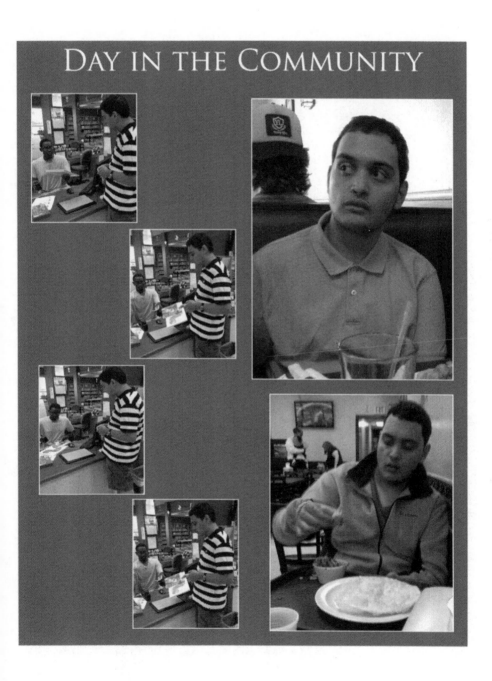

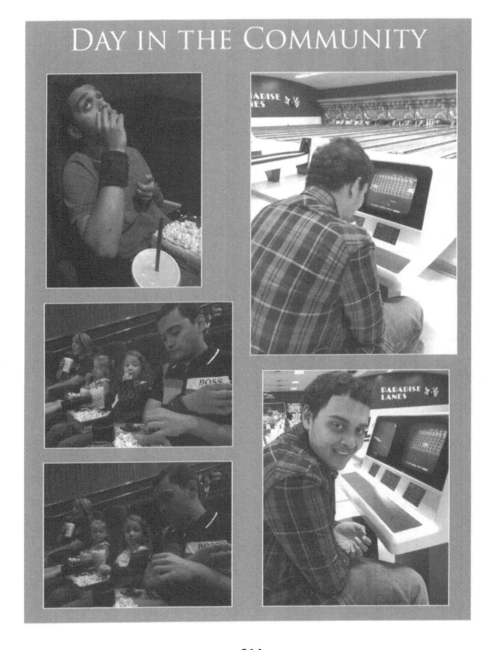

DAY IN THE COMMUNITY

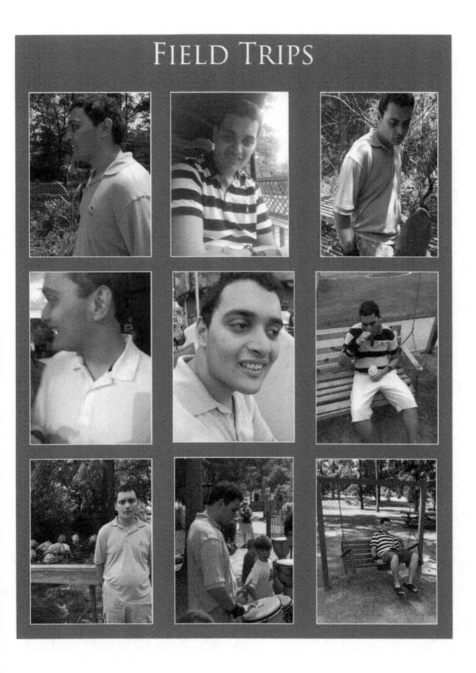

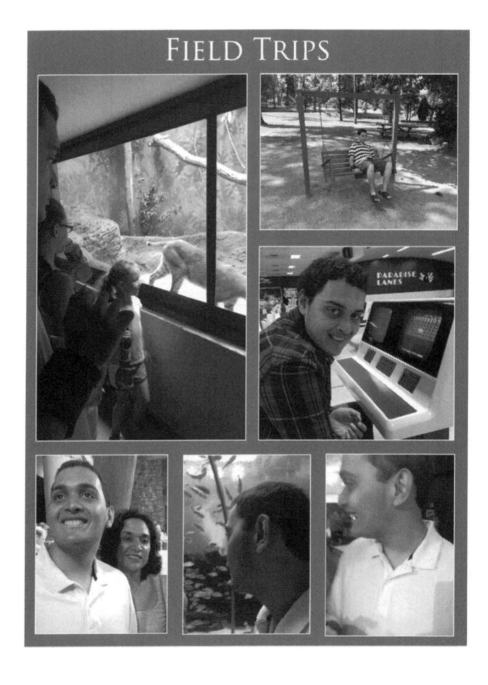

FIELD TRIPS

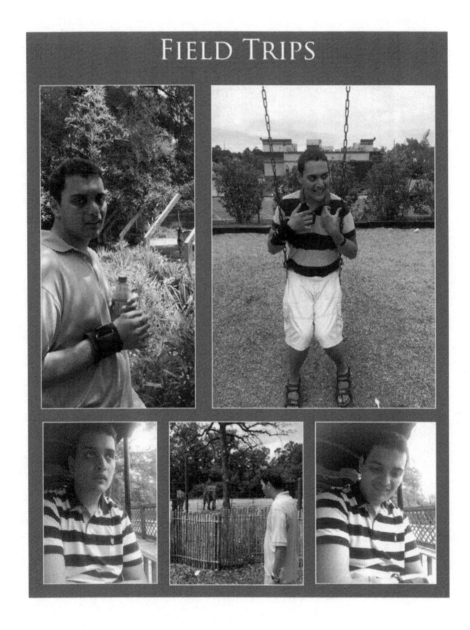

FIELD TRIPS

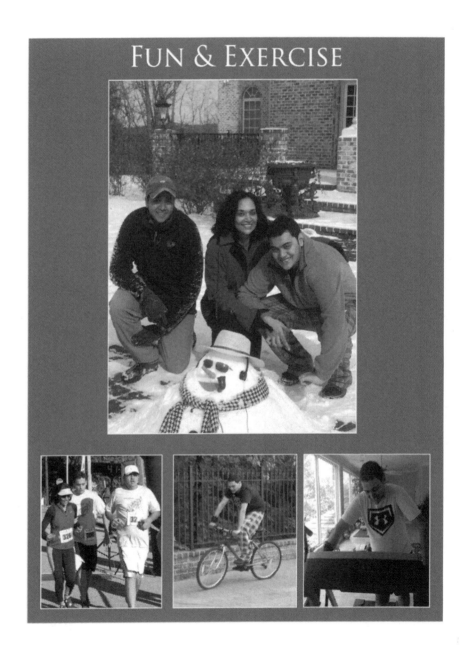

DAILY LIVING SKILLS

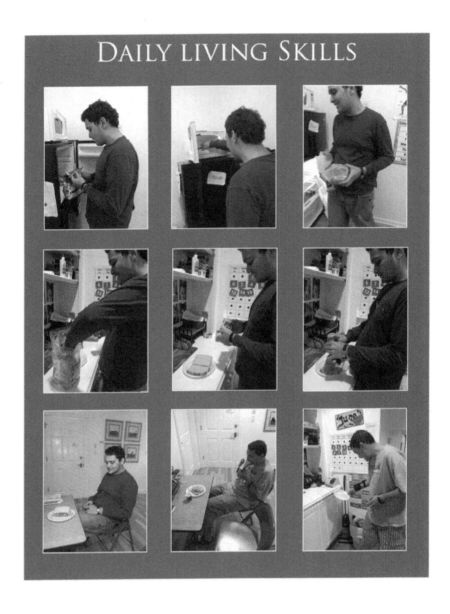

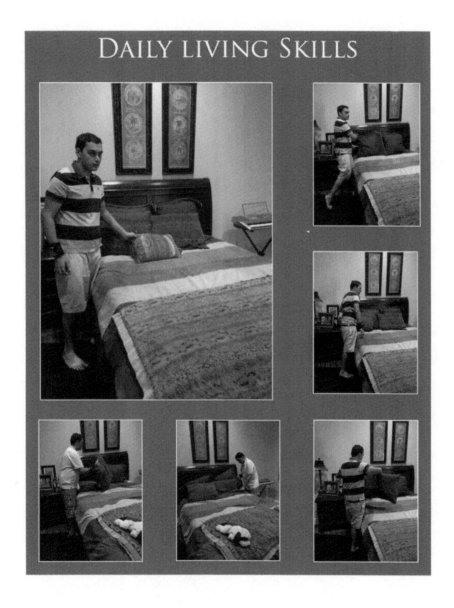

DAILY LIVING SKILLS

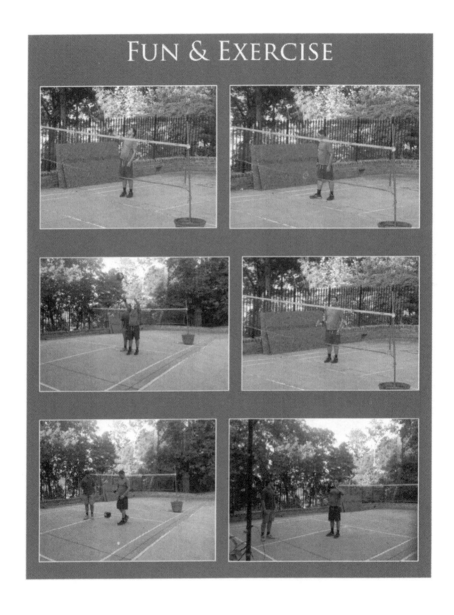

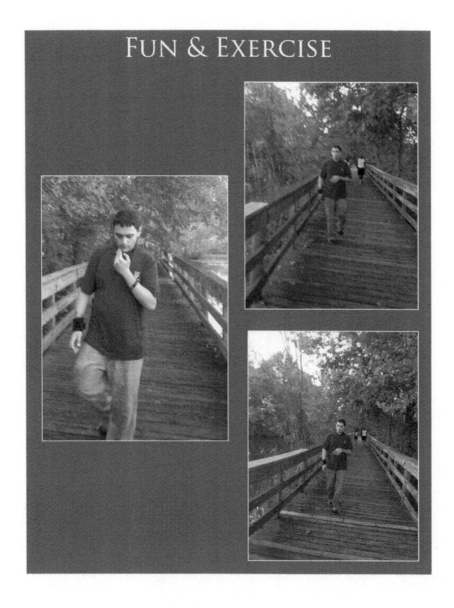

FUN & EXERCISE

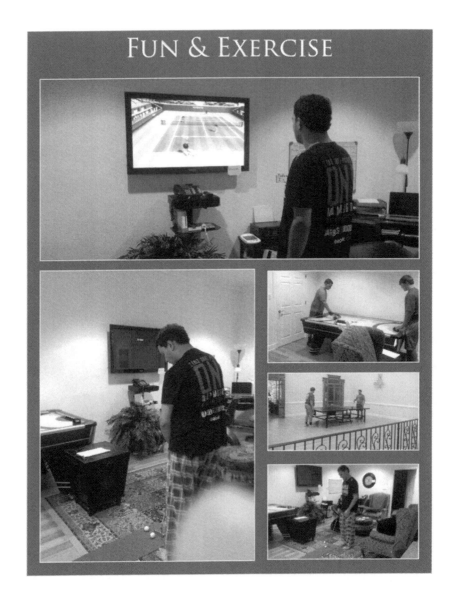

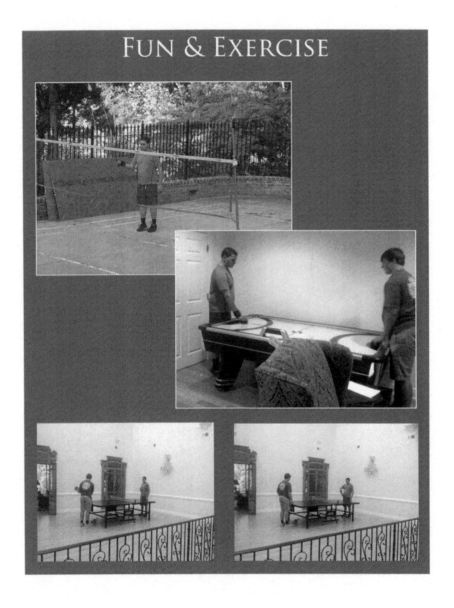

FUN & EXERCISE

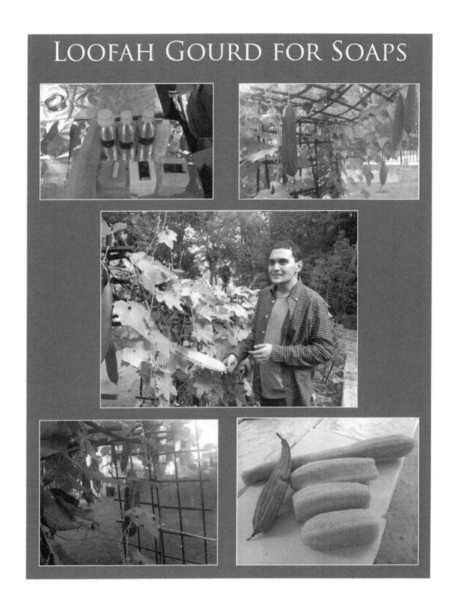

LOOFAH GOURD FOR SOAPS

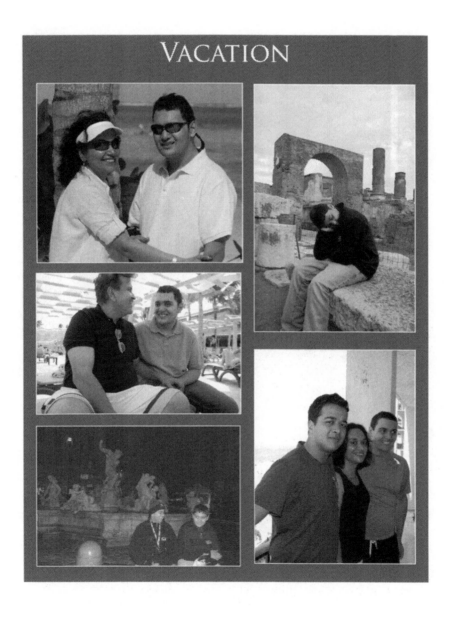

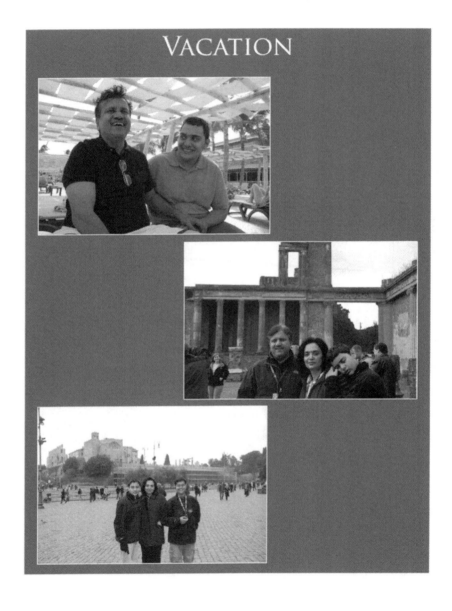

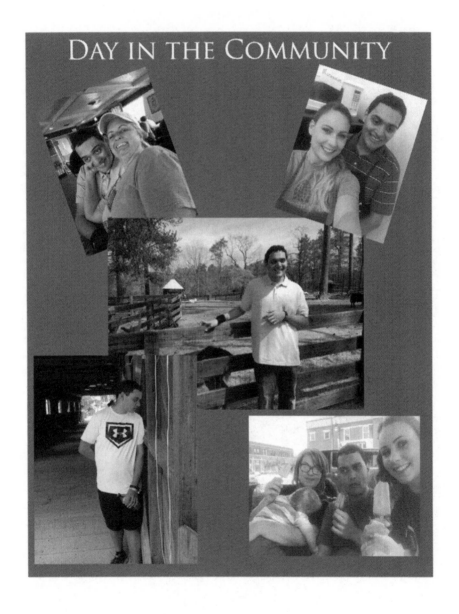

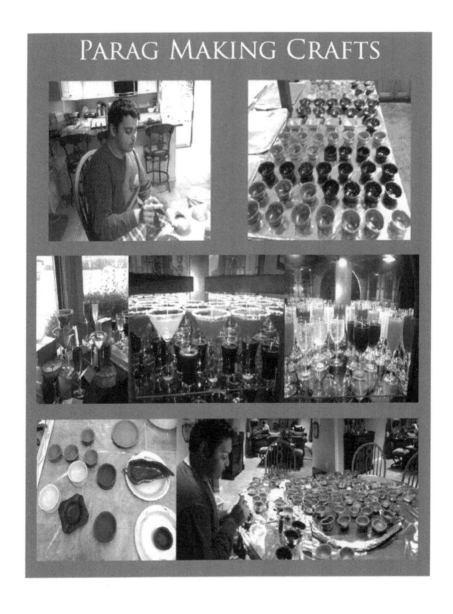

PARAG MAKING CRAFTS

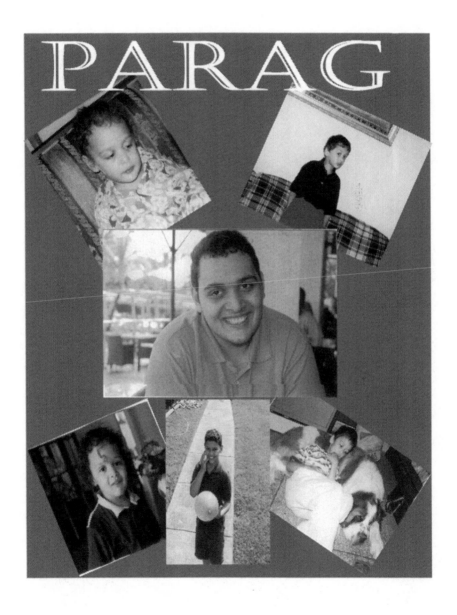

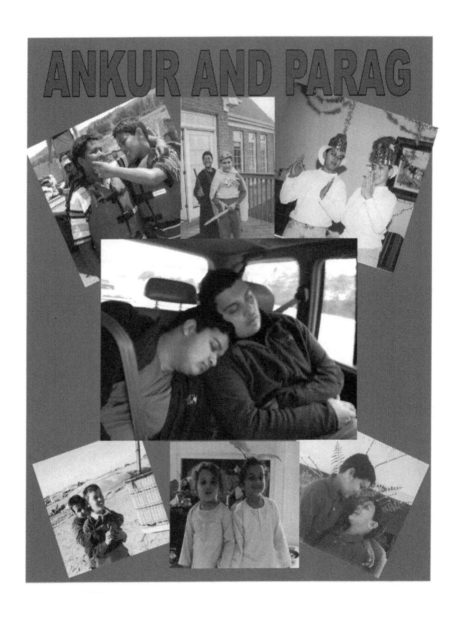

ANKUR AND PARAG

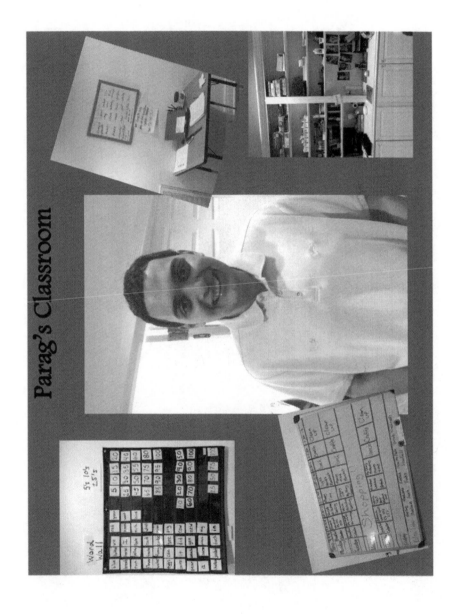

Parag's Classroom

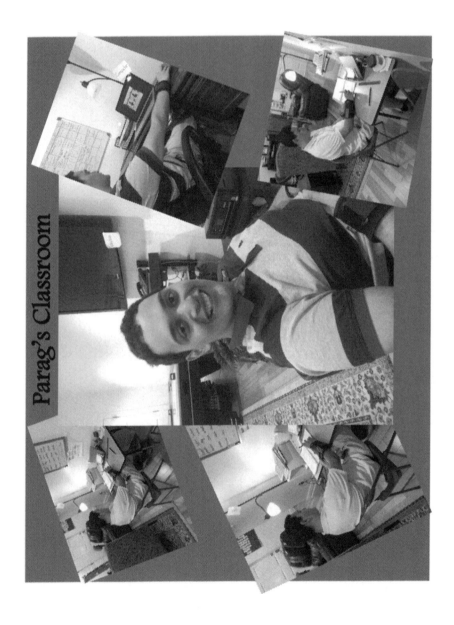

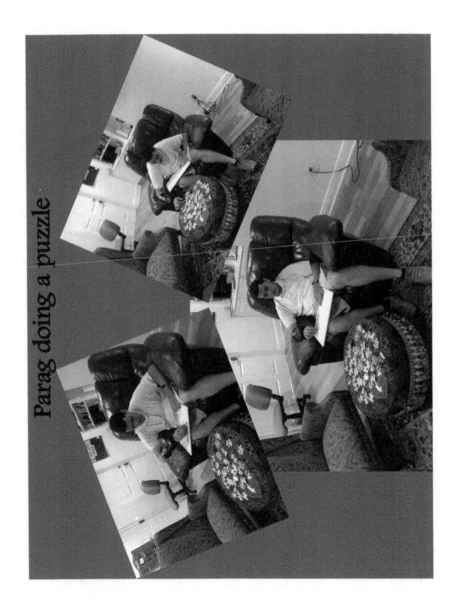

Parag doing a puzzle

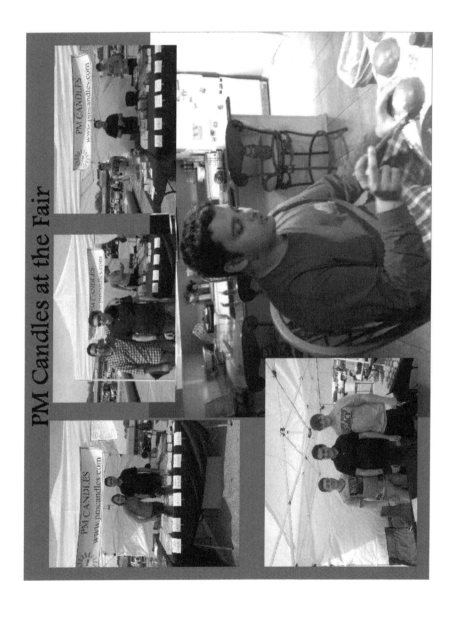

PM Candles at the Fair

Mamta Mishra

References

· Behavioral treatment and normal education and intellectual functioning in young autistic children. Lovaas, o. I. (1987). Journal of Consulting and Clinical Psychology.

· McGee, G.G. Morrier, M.J. & Daly.(1999). An Incidental teaching approach to early intervention for toddlers with autism. JASH, 24 (3), 133-146.

· McLeod, S.A. (2007). Behaviorist Approach. Retrieved from http://www.simplypsychology.org/behaviorism.html

· McLeod, S.A. (2007). Pavlov's Dogs. Retrieved from http://www.simplypsychology.org/pavlov.html

· Mouridsen SE, et al. Mortality and causes of death in autism spectrum disorders: an update. Autism.2008 jul;12(4):403-14

· Pavlov, I.P (1927).Conditioned Reflexes. London: Oxford University Press.

· Shavelle RM, et al. Causes of Death in autism. J Autism Dev Disorder. 2001 Dec; 31(6): 569-76

· Skinner, B.F. (1953). Science and Human Behavior. New York: Macmillan.

· Watson, J.B., & Rayner, R. (1920). Conditioning emotional reactions. Journal of Experimental Psychology, 3.1.pp.1-14.

Mamta Mishra

The Author

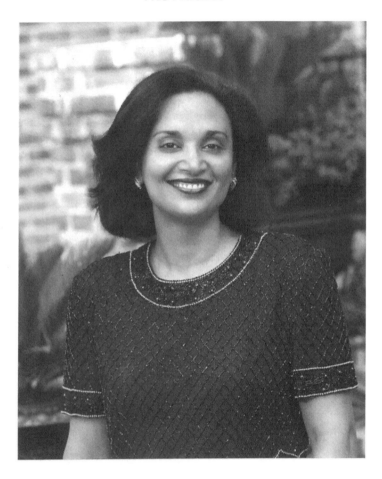

Mamta Mishra was born in India. She did her Masters in English literature from University of Delhi, India and Masters in Special Education from Jacksonville State University, Alabama, U.S.A. Mamta lives in Gadsden, Alabama with her husband, Pranav and two sons, Ankur and Parag. She loves organic gardening, Cross Fit and yoga.

Mamta Mishra

Mamta Mishra

Made in the USA
Lexington, KY
30 May 2018